first place

4health

Bible Study Series

giving Christ
control

Published by Gospel Light
Ventura, California, U.S.A.
www.gospellight.com
Printed in the U.S.A.

Caution: The information contained in this book is intended to be solely for
informational and educational purposes. It is assumed that the First Place 4 Health
participant will consult a medical or health professional before beginning this or
any other weight-loss or physical fitness program.

Library of Congress Cataloging-in-Publication Data
First Place 4 Health Bible study series : giving Christ control.
p. cm. — (First Place 4 Health Bible study series)
ISBN 978-0-8307-5112-9 (trade paper)
1. Trust in God—Christianity—Textbooks. 2. Trust in God—Biblical teaching.
3. Control (Psychology)—Religious aspects—Christianity—Textbooks. 4. Sub-
missiveness—Religious aspects—Christianity—Textbooks. 5. Weight loss—Religious aspects—Christianity—Textbooks. I. First Place 4 Health
(Organization) II. Title: First Place for Health Bible study series.
III. Title: Giving Christ control.
BV4637.F47 2009
231—dc22
2009016636

Rights for publishing this book outside the U.S.A. or in non-English
languages are administered by Gospel Light Worldwide, an international
not-for-profit ministry. For additional information, please visit
www.glww.org, email info@glww.org, or write to Gospel Light Worldwide,
1957 Eastman Avenue, Ventura, CA 93003, U.S.A.

contents

foreword

My introduction to Bible study came when I joined First Place in March 1981. I had been attending church since I was a small child, but the extent of my study of the Bible had been reading my Sunday School quarterly on Saturday night. On Sunday morning, I would listen to my Sunday School teacher as she taught God's Word to me. During the worship service, I would listen to our pastor as he taught God's Word to me. Frankly, the idea of digging out the truths of the Bible for myself had never entered my mind.

Perhaps you are right where I was back in 1981. If so, you are in for a blessing you never dreamed possible. As you start studying the truths of the Bible for yourself through the First Place 4 Health Bible studies, you will see God begin to open your understanding of His Word.

Almost every First Place 4 Health member I have talked with about the program says, "The weight loss is wonderful, but the most important thing I have received from my association with First Place 4 Health is learning to study God's Word." The First Place 4 Health Bible studies are designed to be done on a daily basis. As you work through each day's study (which will take 15 to 20 minutes to complete), you will be discovering the deep truths of God's Word. A part of each week's study will also include a Bible memory verse for the week.

There are many in-depth Bible studies on the market. The First Place 4 Health Bible studies are not designed for the purpose of in-depth study, but are designed to be used in conjunction with the rest of the program to bring balance into your life. Our desire is for each member to begin having a personal quiet time with God each day. This time alone with God should include a time of prayer, Bible reading and Bible study. Having a quiet time is a daily discipline that will bring the rich rewards of balance, which is something we all need.

God bless you as you begin this exciting journey toward a balanced life. God will richly bless your efforts to give Him first place in your life. Remember Matthew 6:33: "But seek first his kingdom and his righteousness, and all these things will be given to you as well."

Carole Lewis, First Place 4 Health National Director

introduction

First Place 4 Health is a Christ-centered health program that emphasizes balance in the physical, mental, emotional and spiritual areas of life. The First Place 4 Health program is meant to be a daily process. As we learn to keep Christ first in our lives, we will find that He is the One who satisfies our hunger and our every need.

This Bible study is designed to be used in conjunction with the First Place 4 Health program but can be beneficial for anyone interested in obtaining a balanced lifestyle. The Bible study has been created in a five-day format, with the last two days reserved for reflection on the material studied. Keep in mind that the ultimate goal of studying the Bible is not only for knowledge but also for application and a changed life. Don't feel anxious if you can't seem to find the *correct* answer. Many times, the Word will speak differently to different people, depending on where they are in their walk with God and the season of life they are experiencing. Be prepared to discuss with your fellow First Place 4 Health members what you learned that week through your study.

There are some additional components included with this study that will be helpful as you pursue the goal of giving Christ first place in every area of your life:

- **Group Prayer Request Form:** This form is at the end of each week's study. You can use this to record any special requests that might be given in class.

- **Leader Discussion Guide:** This discussion guide is provided to help the First Place 4 Health leader guide a group through this Bible study. It includes ideas for facilitating a First Place 4 Health class discussion for each week of the Bible study.

- **Two Weeks of Menu Plans with Recipes:** There are 14 days of meals, and all are interchangeable. Each day totals 1,400 to 1,500 calories and includes snacks. Instructions are given for those who need more calories. An accompanying grocery list includes items needed for each week of meals.

- **First Place 4 Health Member Survey:** Fill this out and bring it to your first meeting. This information will help your leader know your interests and talents.

- **Personal Weight and Measurement Record:** Use this form to keep a record of your weight loss. Record any loss or gain on the chart after the weigh-in at each week's meeting.

- **Weekly Prayer Partner Forms:** Fill out this form before class and place it into a basket during the class meeting. After class, you will draw out a prayer request form, and this will be your prayer partner for the week. Try to call or email the person sometime before the next class meeting to encourage that person.

- **Live It Trackers:** Your Live It Tracker is to be completed at home and turned in to your leader at your weekly First Place 4 Health meeting. The Tracker is designed to help you practice mindfulness and stay accountable with regard to your eating and exercise habits. Step-by-step instructions for how to use the Live It Tracker are provided in the Member's Guide.

- **Let's Count Our Miles!** A worthy goal we encourage is for you to complete 100 miles of exercise during your 12 weeks in First Place 4 Health. There are many activities listed on pages 255-256 that count toward your goal of 100 miles. When you complete a mile of activity, mark off the box listed on the Hundred Mile Club chart located on the inside of the back cover.

- **Scripture Memory Cards:** These cards have been designed so you can use them while exercising. It is suggested that you punch a hole in the upper left corner and place the cards on a ring. You may want to take the cards in the car or to work so you can practice each week's Scripture memory verse throughout the day.

- **Scripture Memory CD:** All 10 Scripture memory verses have been put to music at an exercise tempo in the CD at the back of this study. Use this CD when exercising or even when you are just driving in your car. The words of Scripture are often easier to memorize when accompanied by music.

welcome to
Giving Christ Control

At your first group meeting for this session of First Place 4 Health, you will meet your fellow members, get an overview of your materials and find out what you can expect at weekly meetings. The majority of your class time will be spent learning about the four-sided person concept, the Live It Food Plan, and how change begins from the inside out. You will also have a chance to ask any questions about how to get the most out of First Place 4 Health. If possible, complete the Member Survey on page 205 before your first group meeting. The information that you give will help your leader tailor the next 12 weeks to the needs of the whole group.

Each weekly meeting begins with a weigh-in for members. This will allow you to track your progress over the 12-week session. Your Week One weigh-in/measurement will establish a baseline of comparison so that you can set healthy goals for this session. If you are apprehensive about weighing in every week, talk with your group leader about your concerns. He or she will have some options for you to consider that will make the weigh-in activity encouraging rather than stressful.

The day after your first meeting, begin Week Two of this Bible study. This session, you and your group will study what it means to yield your life to Christ. He's good, He loves you, and He's got great things ahead for you as you continue to follow Him! As you open yourself to the truth of Scripture and share your hopes and struggles with the members of your group during the next 12 weeks, you'll find yourself becoming the healthy child of God you are designed to be!

relying on His goodness

SCRIPTURE MEMORY VERSE
*Restore to me the joy of your salvation
and grant me a willing spirit, to sustain me.*
PSALM 51:12

How much of our lives are truly under our control? Our health? Our finances? Our job? Our family? Living a balanced life is in many ways paradoxical. On the one hand, we want to live with self-control. It is a fruit of the Spirit that is necessary to healthy living, and we want to work and pray consistently to exchange our impulses for the greater good. On the other hand, even when we live with self-control, so much of our lives are *beyond* our control. So much of the time, we can't control what happens around us, to us or to those we love. So what do we do?

That's where we must learn to rely on Christ. God is good. He loves us, and He invites us to live immersed and surrounded by His grace and goodness. Only by consistently yielding ourselves to Him do our lives begin to make sense.

The invitation to give Christ control can seem unnerving at first. Many of us have spent so much time trying to get things under control that it may seem counterintuitive to yield up any of that control to anybody—even God. But giving Christ control never means that we will be *out of control*. Rather, it means that we willfully place the control safely in the hands of God. He is ultimately in charge, and we can always trust Him. The basis for our yielding rests in the knowledge of His righteous character. God is greater than our minds can imagine, and He invites us to rest in Him and dwell securely in His presence.

Yielding our lives to God requires faith and humility. We need to have *faith* in the fact that He has our best plans in mind, and we also need to *humble* ourselves and realize that He knows more than we do. The good news is that when we lower ourselves and demonstrate this type of humility, God lifts us up (see James 4:10). The awesome God of the universe seeks us out and invites us—cloaked in frail humanity as we are—to interface with Him. He invites us to let Him take the lead and be our coach and our guide. He invites us to participate in His plans and is a great respecter of who we are. That's ennobling.

Ultimately, our decision to let Christ take control of our lives is one of worship. By letting Him take the reins, we declare the truth of His righteous character. Whenever we rest in Him, we reflect how great He truly is.

GOD IS ALWAYS GOOD

Day 1

Gracious God, You are always good. I know that this one simple fact is at the core of learning to yield my life to You. Help me to fully grasp this truth today. Amen.

To truly give Christ control of your life, you must be fully convinced of the goodness of God. That one little fact—that God is good—can make all the difference in your faith. After all, if you don't believe that God is good, and *really* good, you will forever be second-guessing your decision to yield your life to Him. You will forever be wondering if you can fully trust Him. And this makes sense, for if God is *not* good, why would you trust Him with your life?

So, how can we truly be convinced of God's goodness? In today's study, we will look at a number of different passages that will provide us with clues about the nature of God. We will begin by looking at the opening story of creation in the Bible.

Begin today's study by reading Genesis 1:4-18. What phrase do you see repeated in these verses?

God made "it" and "it" was good. and He spoke it - making creation personal

What does this tell you about the care that God took in making His creation? What does this imply about the nature of God?

He has high standards and yet made sure everything He created was good. He is good and has good plans for us.

Throughout Scripture, we get other glimpses of this goodness. Read Psalm 31:19 and Psalm 107:1. What does Psalm 107:1 tell us about the type of love God extends to us?

It is a love that never runs out - it is unconditional - I can't exhaust his love - amazing

What images come to mind when you read the words of Psalm 31:19?

towers of gifts - boxes stacked on top of each other of the most amazing gifts

In 1 Timothy 4:4 we read, "For everything God created is good, and nothing is to be rejected if it is received with thanksgiving." This is a profound verse with many far-reaching implications. What do you think it means that everything God created is good?

Are there any exceptions to that rule? Is there anything God has ever created that is *not* good? Why or why not?

what about Satan?

James 1:17 tells us that "every good and perfect gift is from above." What does this tell you about the source of all good things?

from God

James 1:17 also states that every good gift comes "down from the Father of the heavenly lights, who does not change like shifting shadows." What does this passage tell you about the nature of God's love? What similarities do you find between this passage and Psalm 107:1?

it is always constant — the same — not dependant upon me

Is it possible ever to separate what is good from God? Look at David's response in Psalm 16:2. What does this verse tell you?

no -

Let's look at one final example from the book of Exodus 33. When the Israelites were in the desert before they entered the Promised Land, Moses asked God to reveal His glory to him (see v. 18). What was God's response in verse 19?

He chooses to love us me

Now read God's words in Exodus 34:5-7. How can the goodness of God be viewed both as one facet of His glorious nature and the overall summation of His character?

He is just but good, loving, forgiving

God is good. How does this knowledge of His righteous character encourage you to rest in Him? List some practical ways below.

I can trust Him

> *Lord, You are truly good, and good all the time. Help me to never forget this truth. Help me to saturate my mind and heart in it. Amen.*

Day 2

GOD IS GOOD IN GOOD TIMES

Gracious God, when I am in a good season, help me never to forget that You are the origin of all that goodness. Amen.

What's the best thing that's happened to you recently? The birth of a child, a grandchild, a niece or a nephew? A new job or a promotion? Maybe you've reached a goal in personal fitness and you're able to fit into your favorite pair of jeans again. Maybe you've just been through a holiday with friends and loved ones. Or maybe you've been able to spend quality time with a special friend.

We often tend to view life as a struggle, but it's important to remember that there are many good parts to life as well. Seasons of joy really are seasons of worship, because God is the author of all goodness and all goodness comes from Him. Reflecting on our seasons of joy in difficult times can help us remember that we can always rely on Him to pull us through. Remembering His goodness prompts us to continually yield our lives to Him.

For today's study, read John 2:1-11. What would you imagine a Jewish wedding at the time of Christ might be like?

a huge celebration

What does it say about the character of Christ to know that He celebrated at a wedding?

that you enjoy good things - that you enjoy

Jesus instructed servants to fill the stone water jars to the brim with water. Then they took the jars to the master of the banquet, and he tasted what was inside. The water had been miraculously turned into wine. What did the master say about the quality of the wine?

that the best was saved for last - the opposite of what normally happened.

In the culture of that day, wine was a staple of life. Wedding wine would have been good wine to begin with—the type of wine fit for a celebration. This new wine Jesus created was robust, cool, clear and refreshing, the stuff and substance of joy and life. It was the best of wedding wine—the best of the best. What is the significance of Christ using the cold ceremonial water jars for bringing forth what became robust and refreshing?

redemption

In the same way, Christ takes what is spiritually dead and invites us to a transformed way of living. He performs the same miracle with our hearts—turning what was stone cold into joy and life. In what ways have you experienced this goodness of God in your life?

too many to record
—every weakness He can redeem and
bring ministry from - strength

Thinking of times of goodness helps us remember the character of God. How do these remembrances of good times become an encouragement for us to rely on Christ at all times?

Setting up an Ebenezer - because we
are forgetful people—so necessary

As you conclude today's study, think about the best thing that's happened to you recently and how that event, season or experience is a reflection of the goodness of God.

> *Lord, thank You for joy in my life. Each day is a day that You have made. Help me to be joyful and rejoice because of Your goodness. Amen.*

Day 3 GOD IS TRULY GOOD IN UNCLEAR TIMES

Loving God, You are always with me, even when I do not understand Your ways. Help me to sense Your presence and know that You are always there.

It is often easier to understand the goodness of the Lord in the good times than in the bad times. Sometimes when the way is easy, it feels natural for us to praise God and call Him good. However, it is also easy to forget God during such times. There doesn't seem to be a huge need to pray, so we forget to rely on Him or acknowledge that He is the source of *all* the goodness that is in our lives.

At other times when things are tough, we may wonder why we are having to go through such a difficult season. We may have decisions we have to make, and we're just not sure what to do. Or perhaps something happens and we aren't sure why it occurred or what purpose it has in our lives.

Yet it is in these times that we are more likely to turn to God, for we realize that events are beyond our control and we need guidance from the Lord. We have to remember that God is the source of *all* the goodness that is in our lives—both when things are going our way and when they are not.

Today, we are going to be looking at the story of Peter walking on the water. Read Matthew 14:22-32, then answer the following questions.

As the story opens, where are the disciples? Where is Jesus?

they have gone on ahead - in the boat

Jesus is praying - alone

When Jesus saw the disciples were having trouble, He waited until "the fourth watch" (about 3 AM) before walking across the lake to come to them (see v. 25). Why do you think He waited so long?

So they might be extremely aware of their inability to help themselves and their great need for intervention?

Why do you think Jesus sometimes delays when we are going through tough times in our lives?

So we come to the end of ourselves?

What was the disciples' initial response at seeing Jesus walking on the water (see v. 26)?

that He was a ghost

In Isaiah 43:1-4, God tells the Israelites, "When you pass through the waters, I will be with you." How do these words and Jesus' words in Matthew 22:27 help us to not be afraid in unclear times?

our courage can only come from Him and His constant presence.

In verse 28, Peter says, "Lord, if it's you, tell me to come to you on the water." When Jesus tells him to come, he steps out of the boat and walks toward Jesus. He exhibits a lot of faith here, but he also has a problem. What is it?

fear of the unknown - taking his eyes off of His source and focusing on his present situation - loss of perspective

It seems rather amazing that even when Peter is walking on the water—proof that he is moving in the will of Jesus—he begins to doubt! But how do we often do the very same thing when we are faced with a situation in which God calls us to step out in faith?

the reality of the situation can be overwhelming - too much weight to loose, etc.

What was Jesus' response to Peter's sudden call to save him?

immediate - without hesitation

After everyone was safely settled in the boat, the disciples made a declaration to Jesus about who He is. What was that declaration (see v. 32)?

that He truly is the Son of God - Savior - Lord

When the storms of our life come, Christ invites us to remain faithful, fear not, and turn to Him. He is trustworthy. How might this knowledge of God's goodness in the unclear times prompt you to rely on Him more?

remembering His faithfulness helps give me a proper perspective.

Have you had an experience recently (or perhaps are still going through right now) where the way seemed unclear?

Lord, thank You for even the unclear times in my life. Each day is a day that You have made. May I be joyful and rejoice in Your goodness. Amen.

GOD IS GOOD EVEN IN THE HARD TIMES

Day 4

O Gracious God, You are good even when times are hard. Help me to fully grasp this truth even when all around me is painful and dark. Amen.

God is good. Really? Do you really believe that? Always?

It's one thing to talk about the goodness of God when times are joyful, as we discussed on Day Two. It's a bit easier to call God good in the unclear times, as we studied on Day Three. But talking about the goodness of God during the painful times when the path is at its darkest and the way seems too steep to continue—well, that's more difficult.

true

So many times we want to live our lives of faith selectively. For instance, it's easy to live life in light of Psalm 23. We like to think of God as our Shepherd who leads us beside quiet waters and restores our soul. But to get to the banqueting table, we often need to pass through the valley of the shadow—which is part of Psalm 23 as well. To truly grasp this simple yet profound truth—that God is always good—is crucial to living a life resting in Him.

Read Psalm 23. Using the imagery of this psalm, what part of the pathway would you say you are on right now?

not in need of anything - lush meadows and quiet pools to drink from
- the only outstanding issue is my weight

What is one difficult experience you have encountered on your life's pathway? What was your response to God during that time?

Mary - the hardest to understand was our home in Cambridge not selling. - foreclosure after foreclosure = credit ruined
anger - Confusion - Hurt

Did you see the hand of God at work in the situation? If so, describe how God worked in your life during that time.

I did - but mostly as I looked back. Good credit is NOT a need. He provided all our needs - never went hungry or homeless - then provided D.C. = immeasurably more

In John 11:1-43, we find the story of a family who was going through a difficult time. Mary and Martha, two sisters, had a brother named Lazarus who was sick. So the sisters sent word to Jesus saying, "Lord, the one you love is sick" (v. 3). How did Jesus respond (see vv. 4-6)?

He waited - and caused them all to wait, too.

Have you had a situation in your life where it seemed that Jesus was taking a long time to arrive and help you? Describe that time.

again - the Cambridge home situation

God is not lazy or unable to meet your need in a timely way. In fact, He has perfect timing. What do we know about the Lord's perfect timing? (Hint: see Isaiah 49:8.)

Its always perfect

When Lazarus died and Jesus went to see his sisters, what did He tell them about Himself (see v. 25)?

that He was life - those who put their trust in Him would never truly die.

In what ways should His answer have brought comfort to their hearts?

there is more than what we can understand - more - beyond our comprehension.

How does His answer comfort your heart when you are in a hard place?

It all gets redeemed -

The story of Lazarus has a happy ending. Lazarus was resurrected from the dead and was able to continue experiencing life with his sisters, Mary and Martha. However, many stories—both biblical or our own—*don't* have a happy ending. Yet what does Paul tell us in Romans 8:28 we can know even when things don't turn out the way that we had hoped?

all things work together for our good – for those that believe in Him.

Paul's words that "all things work together for good" does not mean that all things will have a way of working out or that we will be free from the effects of sin. It does not mean that random calamity and diseases will never affect us. But it does mean that God knows our every need and cares for us and that He allows suffering to make us more like Christ. He truly does bring about good through the bad things that happen in life, though we may not see how at first. As you conclude today's study, think about how this truth of God's character can help you learn to rely on God even when the way is difficult.

Gracious God, You know our every need, and You care for us. I know that one day everything will be made right because You are a God of justice. Help me to understand this truth and always live in light of it. Amen.

Day 5 — GOD IS ALWAYS GOOD IN OUR LIVES

O Gracious God, what a joy it is when we know that we can always rely on You. You are good and You are in our lives. Amen.

What does the word "goodness" truly mean? We might talk about a good car, or a good ice cream cone, or say we're doing "good" in answer to every general salutation. The word in English can be so broadly applied as to mean everything and nothing.

The English word "good" actually evolved out of the word for God. The expression "goodbye" is a contraction of the phrase "God be with you." From its fundamental roots in our language, we have a basic association of God and "good." Interestingly, the Bible says that God's goodness is available to us through the power of His Holy Spirit. In

Romans 15:14, Paul indicates that it's possible for people to be filled with God's goodness.

Have you ever thought about yourself in those terms? When you know that God is working within you and you know that He is good, it can give you greater reason to rely on Him fully. Today, we will look at a few Scriptures that show this idea in action.

"Goodness," as defined by Scripture, is the state of those who have received the righteousness of Christ and have become part of the kingdom of God. Read Titus 3:3-7. What is it that makes any person good?

the Holy Spirit's washing - inside and out.

In 2 Corinthians 13:5, Paul writes, "Do you not realize that Christ Jesus is in you?" What might this mean in the context of goodness?

His very character is good - therefore, because of Christ's indwelling - "I am good" - do good, etc.

In Philippians 2:13, Paul writes, "It is God who works in you to will and to act according to his good purpose." What does it mean to have God at work in you?

being submitted to the Holy Spirit - allowing Him to lead - listening; acting on what we hear

Read Romans 15:14. Have you ever thought of yourself as being filled with God's goodness? What might God's goodness in your life look like?

Sometimes - I get a lot of credit for doing extraordinary things - I KNOW He is the source of every bit of that, but I do forget in other ways - when I'm struggling with sin.

In Ephesians 5:18, Paul encourages us to be filled with the Spirit, or under the Spirit's control. Praying for the filling of the Spirit works in conjunction with our obedience to God's commands. This combination of prayer and obedience allows the Spirit freedom to work within us. How can you have confidence that your life is filled with goodness?

I've experienced it

How can you have confidence every day in your First Place 4 Health journey that what you say, do, think, feel and even remember is good—or at least filtered through what is good?

that's harder for me - I'm an "in the moment" person. In the moment I have no doubt but in general I struggle to remember that.

Lord God Almighty, thank You for Your Holy Spirit, who is active and involved in my life. Thank You for the confidence that Christ lives within me and that I have the power every day to live in the Spirit's control. Amen.

Day 6

REFLECTION AND APPLICATION

Thank You, God, that You are good, truly good, and good all the time. Your goodness is the foundation of my reliance on You. Amen.

"God is good." Such a simple phrase, and yet it is so profound in its implications. God is good in His entirety. In fact, the goodness of God is a character trait that applies to every other attribute He possesses. God is all good, all the time, and everything about Him is good. God's holiness is good. God's righteousness is good. Even God's wrath is good. There is nothing about Him that is anything otherwise.

Similarly, there is nothing God purposes for His children that is not good. God gives to His children only that which is good, and He withholds nothing good from them. He is at work in His children' good and everything that He creates and accomplishes is for th _____ fit. God is good all the time. Always. Spend some time today just reflecting on the goodness of God.

God, thank You for this attribute You possess of always being good.
Help me to remember that one fact about You—Your goodness. Amen.

REFLECTION AND APPLICATION

Day
7

Lord, help me to immerse my life in the truth of Your goodness.
Allow me to see how You have always been good to me in the past
and help me to trust that You will take care of my future. Amen.

Today, spend some time journaling about your life. Write down some significant events that have occurred in your life, both good and bad. Then, beside each event, write down a phrase to help you filter all of your life through God's goodness, such as "God is good," or "yet I know God is good," or "in spite of this, God is good."

Now go through each of the items in your list and fill in the words after the "because." As you do this, think about how God worked through the situation and revealed His hand in your life. Was there something you felt He wanted you to learn from the experience? Did you find yourself getting closer to God through the situation? Did He demonstrate to you that you could always rely on Him in any circumstance? How exactly did He show His goodness to you on a personal level?

Once you have completed this exercise, spend some time in prayer thanking God that even in the good times and the bad, He is always with you. He is truly always good.

Lord, not everything in this world is good, yet Your goodness
extends to everything. Help me to see my life in light of Your
goodness. I place my life in Your hands. Amen.

Group Prayer Requests

4 first place
health

Today's Date: _____

Name	Request

Results

_____

_____

_____

_____

_____

convinced of
His love

SCRIPTURE MEMORY VERSE
May the God of hope fill you with all joy and peace as you trust in him, so that you may overflow with hope by the power of the Holy Spirit.

ROMANS 15:13

In addition to the goodness of God, there's another foundational truth about God's righteous character that is necessary for us to grasp in order for us to truly live our lives yielded to Him. It's God's love. This is the idea that God, by grace, is favorably inclined toward us. After all, if God were good but indifferent toward us, why would we rely on Him? But if He is good and cares about us, then we can confidently place our lives in His hands.

Look at the memory verse this week. In this passage, Paul is praying that believers will understand the righteous character of God and live with full dependence on Him. When we yield control to God and allow Him to work within us, He fills our lives with benefits such as joy, peace and hope. Each of these comes as a result of God's love. He invites us to live lives immersed and surrounded by His grace, goodness and love. Only by consistently yielding ourselves to Him do our lives make sense.

As mentioned last week, our decision to let Christ take control of our lives is ultimately one of worship. By letting Him take the reins of our lives, we are declaring the truth of God's righteous character. Whenever we rest in Him, we reflect how great He truly is. This week, we will take a look at this awesome love that God has for us.

GOD DEFINES LOVE

Gracious God, You are love. This truth is at the core of learning to yield to You. Help me to grasp that You are the very definition of love itself. Amen.

When John wrote in his first letter that "God is love," he was not telling us that God is some nebulous, warm fuzzy feeling of love. Neither was he or any of the other writers who penned the Scriptures saying that by practicing our limited form of human love we will find God. Rather, when we read that God is love, it means that God *defines* love.

Now, He doesn't define it like *Webster's* might define something. No, He is the definition of love itself. He is the author of love. He created it and embodies it. In fact, His very nature is love. There is no such thing as love without God, and as hard as we might try, we cannot define it outside of Him. His love is unconditional and sacrificial, and it's not based on feelings. God's love is not a "strong affection for another arising out of kinship or personal ties," as *Webster's* defines love.[1] It is more.

To understand what true love is and to be able to truly love others, we must first know God, and we can only do that by having a close personal relationship with Him. How do we develop a personal relationship with God? By putting our faith in Jesus Christ, who was God's sacrifice of love for us. When we know this love of God and understand that God is love, we can then rely on Him completely.

Read 1 John 4:7-8. How does God define love?

_____

_____

_____

One of the best-known verses in the Bible is John 3:16. In this verse, how does God define His love?

_____

_____

_____

God proved His love not by giving us a gift-wrapped present but by taking on the form of a man, coming to earth, and laying down His life so that we can spend eternity with Him. How does knowing this prompt you further to yield your life to Him?

_____

_____

_____

_____

Another great verse about God's love is found in Romans 5:8. In this amazing passage, we find that God places no conditions on His love for us. He doesn't say, "As soon as you clean up your act, I'll love you," or, "I'll sacrifice my Son if you promise to love Me." Actually, we find just the opposite. His love is *unconditional*. He died for us while we were still unlovable sinners. We didn't have to get cleaned up first, and we didn't have to make any promises to God before we could experience His love.

Read Psalm 86:5. What does this tell us about the extent of God's love?

_____

_____

_____

_____

One definition of "abounding" is "to be fully supplied."[2] What does the fact that God's love is "abounding" mean in your life?

_____

_____

_____

Now look at Psalm 118. What phrase do you see repeated in this psalm?

_____

_____

_____

Conclude today's study by spending some time considering the love that God, through His gift of Jesus, has shown to you. You may want to complete the following sentences:

Because I know that Jesus loves me, I can . . .

_____

_____

_____

The best example I've ever seen of Christ's love in my own life is . . .

_____

_____

_____

I will take the following action in response to God's love . . .

_____

_____

_____

Oh Lord, You are what love is all about. Help me to never forget this truth. Help me to saturate my mind and heart in with Your love. Help me learn to rely on You. Amen.

Day 2 — GOD'S LOVE IS THE GREATEST

Lord, Your love is everything. All I have and all I am is nothing without Your love. Help me to understand the depth of Your love today. Amen.

We hear a lot about love today. It's a word that's used everywhere. We love oranges. We love cats (or not). We love our friends. We love God. And we know that God loves us. But what does that exactly mean—that God *loves* us? In learning to rely on God fully, it's helpful to dive into an extended definition of the love that Christ has for us. And perhaps the single greatest extended biblical definition of love is found in 1 Corinthians 13. You've probably heard this passage before—parts of it are often read at weddings. But have you ever read this passage through the paradigm of God's love for us? We'll take a look at this passage today.

What are some of the gifts and "good deeds" that Paul lists in verses 1-3?

_____

_____

_____

What does Paul say about the value of these things if we do not have the love of God?

_____

_____

_____

Read verses 4-7. Every time you see the word "love" or "it" referring to love, say the word "God." Now, apply those verses to your own life using the sentences below:

Because God is patient, I know He is patient toward me when I . . .

_____

_____

_____

Because Christ keeps no record of wrongs, I know that when I make a mistake . . .

_____

_____

_____

Because God does not rejoice in unrighteousness, I know that He will . . .

_____

_____

_____

In verse 8, Paul says that God's love never fails. How can this knowledge help you learn to rely on Him more fully?

_____

_____

_____

Read verses 9-12. How do increased spiritual maturity, God's love, and relying on Christ fit together?

_____

_____

_____

Now write down one descriptive word to help you remember the extent of Christ's love for you. For example: "Christ's love is *eternal*" or, "Christ's love is *complete*." How will remembering this word change your life?

_____

_____

_____

Oh Lord, Your love is amazing. Help me to never forget this about You.
Your love continues forever and ever. Thank You for your love. Amen.

Day 3 — GOD'S LOVE IS SCANDALOUS

Lord, Your love extends to all. It extends and extends and extends.
Your love brought a cross to Your Son. Your love saves the world. Amen.

In her memoir *Finding Martha's Place*, Alabama restaurateur Martha Hawkins tells the story about founding her restaurant on the principles of the "scandalous terms of grace."[3] One of the ways she put this decision into action was to constantly hire workers from varied backgrounds in order to offer them a second chance at life. For instance, she would often hire former drug addicts, women recently released from the nearby prison, and anyone else who was generally down on his or her luck.

Martha tells about one such worker named Richard who was a former drug addict but was trying to make a clean break of things. Richard did okay in the job for a while, but then he got off track and stole Martha's car, lied to her and robbed her restaurant so that he could buy crack. Richard was arrested and sent to jail, where he underwent a drug program that enabled him to be released. There was only one problem: Richard needed to have a job lined up in order for him to be released. Martha was the only potential employer he knew, so he called her from jail and asked for his old job back.

What would Martha do? She fully believed in giving people second chances, but this was Richard's fourth or fifth or sixth. There was a strong possibility he would make the same poor decisions in the future. In making her decision, Martha was reminded of the story of the prodigal son. It's a familiar story to many, but let's take a look at it together.

Read Luke 15:11-32. What does the younger son ask of his father?

_____

_____

_____

In Jewish culture, for a young man to ask for a share of his inheritance before his father was deceased was the equivalent of wishing his father was already dead. This request was not simply a blunder on the young man's part but was also a willful and deliberate swipe at his father. What happens to the young man next (see vv. 13-16)?

_____

_____

_____

What realization does the young man eventually make (see vv. 17-20)?

_____

_____

_____

Do you think this realization was an indication of true repentance? Was the young man truly changed at this point? Why or why not?

_____

_____

_____

Once the young man comes to his senses, he decides to return to his father. What is significant about the phrase, "while he was still a long way off" in verse 20 as it relates to his father's reception of him?

_____

_____

_____

What might be significant about this phrase as it applies to your personal relationship with God?

_____

_____

_____

It has been said that in Jewish culture, wealthy and powerful men never ran. It was considered embarrassing, even disgraceful, for a grown man to be seen running.[4] Yet in verse 20, we see the father sprinting to greet his wayward son. What does this tell you about God's love for us?

_____

_____

_____

How would you characterize the father's words to his older son in verses 31-32? Describe God's love in relation to what the father tells the older son about his feelings and actions toward the younger son.

_____

_____

_____

As you conclude today's study, look back on your First Place 4 Health journey. In what ways might you have strayed from what God has called you to do in terms of maintaining a balanced and healthy lifestyle? Have you surrendered control of that area of your life to God?

_____

_____

_____

_____

God the Father knows our struggles and is always ready and willing to help us get back on track. Remember, He is the very definition of love itself, and He can't wait to coming running to us when we acknowledge our need for Him. Spend a few moments today thanking God for being such a loving Father and for His incredible mercy and grace.

> *Lord, Your love is often scandalous. You give second and third and fifth and eightieth chances. Thank You for Your extreme love. Amen.*

RESTING IN GOD'S LOVE

Day 4

> *Heavenly Father, I want to cease striving, stop running, stop chasing and simply know that You are God. Amen.*

Immersing ourselves in the reality of God's love is vital to our learning to give Christ control over our lives. When we know God and sense His love, we can rest in Him. We don't need to be restless for the next conquest, striving to gain what is beyond our reach and gripping tightly to that which is fleeting. God invites us to lean against His love. He invites us to relax and let go.

The Bible gives us a brief but beautiful picture of love in Psalm 131. In just three verses, David shows us what it's like to rest securely in the will of God. He offers us a picture of contentment in spite of contrary tendencies. Read this psalm, and then linger over the verses for a while. You might want to even read these three verses several times slowly.

How would you describe the mood, tone and feel of this psalm?

_____

_____

_____

What is significant about the lowly place the psalmist has taken? Why is it important that humility is shown as leading toward rest?

_____

_____

_____

_____

In verse 2, the psalmist says that he has stilled and quieted his soul "like a weaned child with its mother." How does a breast-fed child respond when he is first given a bottle?

_____

_____

_____

After the child is fully weaned, how does he act?

_____

_____

_____

After a while, the child becomes content with the bottle. In the same way, the psalmist indicates that he was once ambitious and restless—he wanted to walk in ways that were beyond him—but now he is filled with quietness and contentment. In light of this psalm, what is the foundation for victory over feverish cravings and ambitions (see v. 3)?

_____

_____

_____

To conclude today's study, write out a few practical applications to this psalm. You can use the following prompts:

Lord, I've been ambitious for _____,
but now, let me simply put my hope in You by yielding this area of my life to You.

Lord, You know my craving for _____,
but now, let me simply put my hope in You by yielding this area of my life to You.

Lord, let me be like that child who once struggled with his mother but is now at rest with her. Restore Your peace and harmony to me. Amen.

THE "GROAN" OF GOD'S LOVE
Day 5

Jesus, thank You for Your work on the cross. You have bridged the gap between God and man. You have made a way for us to have intimate access to the Father. Thank You for this love. Amen.

Life can throw a constant stream of hardships our way. But how often do we stop to consider that because of God's perfect love for us, these hardships could actually be part of His perfect plan for our lives? Our task is neither to embrace these hardships nor to seek more of them. Rather, our task is simply to rely on God and know His love for us in the midst of those hardships. In difficult times, our invitation is to press in closer to the Lord.

The Bible tells us that we have a constant ally through any difficulty, someone who constantly helps us in our weaknesses. As children of God, the Holy Spirit lives inside of us. Part of His job is to "translate" our prayers to the Father. Some of these prayers may even be prayed without words. This is just another example of God's love for us: intimacy. God knows us through and through, even in our most difficult times, and He is always ready to be our rock and our source of comfort. Let's look at a key passage today that illustrates this idea.

Read Romans 8:18-28. Paul states that our present sufferings are far outweighed by the glory that will be revealed in us. This future glory is so great that present sufferings are insignificant by comparison. To what kind of glory is Paul referring? (Hint: see 2 Corinthians 4:17-18.)

_____

_____

_____

In verse 20, Paul states that "creation was subjected to frustration." This refers to the effects of the original fall of mankind—effects that include the decay and frailty that can be found throughout the world. How have you experienced this sense of frustration in your own life?

_____

_____

_____

In verse 23, Paul writes that we are all eagerly awaiting our adoption as sons. This verse might seem paradoxical at first. We know from the Bible that God has given us His spirit of sonship (see Romans 8:15) and that we are already children of God (see Galatians 4:6-7). But in this passage, what Paul is saying is that as believers, we are eagerly awaiting the completion of this "adoption" process, or the experience of a full release from the effects of sin. This will happen sometime in the future, in the day when all things are made right by God. How might this knowledge of a future release from the effects of sin prompt us to rely on Him more now?

_____

_____

_____

_____

In verse 26, Paul states that the Spirit helps us in our weaknesses by interceding for us with "groans that words cannot express." The Greek word for "weakness" (*astheneia*) used in this verse may include any physical, emotional, spiritual or mental weakness. The word translated as "groaning" (*stenagmos*) connotes a picture of someone helping another by carrying a heavy load. The idea is that the Holy Spirit carries our loads. What "load" are you currently carrying?

_____

_____

_____

_____

The love of God is an intimate love. God does not expect us to figure out life all on our own. He invites us to let Him carry our burdens. How will this knowledge prompt you to rely on Him more?

_____

_____

_____

_____

Oh Lord, let me rest in the knowledge that You love me so much that Your Holy Spirit groans with my burdens. I rest in You. Amen.

REFLECTION AND APPLICATION

Day
6

God, You love us deeply, purely and scandalously. You love us more than we will ever know. Thank You so much for this truth. Amen.

A story is told of a young man who once wanted to take a cruise aboard a luxury liner. He didn't have much money, but he saved and saved for months until finally he had enough to purchase his passage. The young man knew that he didn't have enough money for meals, so he packed some bread and cheese.

The young man enjoyed the cruise, but he couldn't help feeling envious when he saw all the other passengers eating in the dining rooms and banquet halls in the ship. After two weeks, the man's bread and cheese began to mold, and he was hungry. Finally, a crewmember noticed his state and approached him to ask if anything was wrong. The young man, slightly embarrassed, explained that he did not have enough money to buy food. It was then that the crewmember informed the man that all the food was included in the price of the ticket.

Sometimes, we are like this young man. God has invited us to live immersed and surrounded by His grace, goodness and love. He calls us to surrender our lives to Him and come to His banquet table. Yet we often choose to hold on to that with which we are familiar instead of yielding our lives completely to Him. When we do, we miss out on all the blessings He has planned for us.

God is the embodiment of love. When we know and experience this love and understand the righteous character of God, we can live with full dependence on Him. By letting Him take the reins of our lives, we can declare the truth of God's righteous character. Whenever we rest in Him, we can reflect how great He truly is and bring glory to His name.

So today, spend some time reflecting on the love of God. You can use the following prompts below and fill in your answers, or you can write your thoughts in your prayer journal.

Because God loves me, I want to thank Him for . . .

_____

_____

The one thing that consistently reminds me of God's love in my life is . . .

_____

_____

Because I know God has a plan and a purpose for my life, I can confidently say . . .

_____

_____

Lord, I want to partake in the blessings You have in store for me. Help me to release control of my life and experience Your amazing love. Amen.

REFLECTION AND APPLICATION

*Lord, You are the author of love, the creator of love, and You are
always loving. Thank You for being all about love. Amen.*

Similar to what we did last week, spend some time today with paper
and pen and journal about your life. Write down some of the significant events that have taken place, both good and bad, and then beside
each incident write a phrase or two that will help you filter what has occurred through the lens of God's love. Some examples to help get you
started are given below.

I don't know what I want to do for a career. *But I know that God loves me because . . .*

I often struggle with food, and I know that I still need to live my life in balance. *Yet I
know that God is love because . . .*

I was so worried about that situation with my friend, but I see how God did a dramatic
work in her life. *This shows me that God is love because . . .*

I am so thankful for my spouse. *I can tell that God truly loves me because . . .*

Just as you did last week, go through each of the items and fill in the
words after the "because." Once you have done this, go over each item
and say a prayer of praise to God for demonstrating His love in the
good times, the bad times, and even in the uncertain times.

*Lord, You are a loving God. You care for me always. Help me see my life in
light of Your love. My life is in Your hands. Amen.*

Notes

1. "love," *Merriam-Webster Unabridged Dictionary* (Springfield, MA: Merriam-Webster, Inc., 2008).
2. "abounding," *The American Heritage Dictionary of the English Language*, Fourth Edition (New York: Houghton Mifflin Company, 2006).
3. Martha Hawkins with Marcus Brotherton, *Finding Martha's Place* (New York: Simon and Schuster, release date 2010).
4. Gerald A. Arbuckle and Jean Vanier, *Laughing with God* (Collegeville, MN: Liturgical Press, 2008), p. 36.

Group Prayer Requests

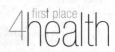

Today's Date: _____

Name	Request

Results

_____

_____

_____

_____

_____

yielding to
His glory

SCRIPTURE MEMORY VERSE
*Finally, brothers, whatever is true, whatever is noble,
whatever is right, whatever is pure, whatever is lovely,
whatever is admirable—if anything is excellent
or praiseworthy—think about such things.*
PHILIPPIANS 4:8

When learning to give Christ control of our lives, the place to start is with God Himself. That's what we've been doing so far—studying the righteous character of a holy, majestic, good and loving God. When we know God—*truly* know Him—and know what He is like, we will be much more intrinsically inclined to put our full trust in Him. God can be trusted with *all* we yield to Him.

But what do we do once we are convinced of God's righteous character? The next step is as simple—and as difficult—as making a decision. The next step in the yielding process is that we decide to give Christ control over our lives. We willfully and purposefully set our lives in His hands. It's a choice we make in prayer, and then our actions follow that choice.

The decision first begins in the mind. We mentally choose to rest in Him. Now, instead of thinking of that decision as a difficult one to make, let's approach it from the standpoint of God's glory. God is the sum total of all truth and beauty anywhere. God is wondrous, majestic, glorious and amazing. When we fill our minds with His glory, we are that much more inclined to choose to follow Him wholeheartedly. Following

God is in our best interest. When we approach it from that standpoint, it's an easier decision to make and continue making.

In this week's study, we will examine how to begin to "think about such things" that our memory verse describes: things that are true, noble, right, pure, lovely, admirable, excellent and praiseworthy.

Day 1 — A MAJESTIC DRAW

God, You are the author and creator of all the truth and beauty that exists. Help me to constantly fix my eyes, mind and heart on You. Amen.

Sometimes when people think about an eternity with Christ, they think that it will be boring. "Imagine, just sitting around on clouds all day playing harps and singing praise songs—that'll soon get old," they say, or words to that effect. But when we truly understand who God is and what being in His presence is like, we realize that nothing could be farther from the truth.

Think of anything good or joyful or fun or majestic or exciting on earth. God is better. That simple truth should be so powerful in our lives: God is better than anything we can imagine. The great theologian Jonathan Edwards once said, "He is indeed possessed of infinite majesty, to inspire us with reverence and adoration; yet that majesty need not terrify us, for we behold it blended with humility, meekness, and sweet condescension." God is all goodness, all joyfulness, all fun, all majesty, all excitement. Being in God's presence is far from boring. When we know what God is truly like, our decision to yield our lives to Him is a natural following. Let's look at this idea more closely.

Read Psalm 19:1-6. How is the glory of the Lord described in this passage?

_____

_____

_____

Read Psalm 27:1-8. How does fear often keep us from giving God control over our lives?

_____

_____

_____

_____

What does David say about God's character in these verses that allows us to set our minds at ease?

_____

_____

_____

What is David's one desire (see v. 4)? What are some practical ways we can have this same desire?

_____

_____

_____

_____

In the present day, what might it look like, in a practical way, to seek the Lord (see vv. 7-8)?

_____

_____

_____

_____

Turn to Hebrews 12:1-3. What does it mean to consistently "fix our eyes on Jesus"? What are some practical examples of how we can do this?

_____

_____

_____

_____

Think about all the things on earth you can that you can describe as being true, noble, right, pure, lovely, great or majestic. God is better. God is the epitome of all greatness, glory and truth. As you conclude today's study, spend some time meditating on this fact—that the beauty of God is better than anything you can imagine. To what extent do you think you truly know this truth, feel it in your heart and live it out?

> *Lord, You are better than anything I can imagine. Thank You that You are all goodness and truth and beauty and glory. Amen.*

Day 2

THINK ON THESE THINGS

Lord, it is always my desire to think about what is noble, true, excellent and praiseworthy, but often that is not the first place my mind goes. Help me today to yield control of my mind to You so that You can renew my thinking.

In our Scripture memory verse for this week, Philippians 4:8, Paul talks about giving Christ control by willfully thinking about good things. As we learned yesterday, God is the epitome of all good things. Thus, one great way to continually give Christ control over our thoughts is to willfully think about God—to fix our minds on Christ, and saturate our heads with all that is noble, true, excellent and praiseworthy.

Of course, this concept of what we willfully fill our minds with has a dangerous side as well. As Ralph Waldo Emerson once said, "Beware of what you set your mind on, for that you will surely become." Our actions begin in our minds and hearts. Behavior often starts by imagining an action, or at least leaning toward it. Then, when our minds have acquiesced to that thought, we begin to act in that manner. As people called to follow Christ and live balanced lives, we cannot afford to allow thoughts to race through our minds unchecked. We must assume responsibility for our thoughts, continually giving them over to Christ and filtering them through His righteousness.

As you begin today's study, consider this idea that behavior begins in the mind. What examples have you seen of this in your own life, or in the lives of others?

_____

_____

_____

_____

Read 1 Corinthians 14:20. What are some practical examples of how we can be "adults" in our thinking?

_____

_____

_____

_____

Read Romans 13:14. How does this verse encourage us to give Christ control over our thoughts?

_____

_____

_____

Now turn to 2 Corinthians 10:5. What does Paul mean when he says that we take every thought captive?

_____

_____

_____

Finally, look up 1 John 4:15-16. How might relying on God's love help us in the area of our thought life?

_____

_____

_____

Giving this area of our lives over to Christ—our thoughts—can be difficult. It is easy to focus on the negatives when something happens that we did not plan, and soon we are not thinking about whatever is noble, true, excellent and praiseworthy . . . but on *just the opposite.* Consider the journey that you have taken in First Place 4 Health so far. What area of your thought life do you still most need to give Christ control over?

_____

_____

_____

_____

Fortunately, we read in Romans 12:2 that we can be transformed by the renewing of our minds. As we submit the control of our thought life to God and train ourselves to think on Him when we encounter difficulties, He can begin the process of transforming our thoughts. When our thoughts are transformed, a change in our behaviors will follow. It's a process, and change may not always come immediately, but if we continually submit the control of our minds over to God, change will occur.

> *Lord, help me to captive every thought. Let me fill my mind with the beauty of Your righteous character and all the goodness that flows from You. Amen.*

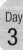

Day 3

THE BATTLE FOR RIGHT AND PURE

Jesus Christ, I exalt Your name. Help me to focus my minds on what is right and pure. You are a beautiful God, and I honor You. Amen.

The battle for our minds is a spiritual one. We must willfully choose each day to take our thoughts captive and make them obedient to Christ. Fortunately, we have the Holy Spirit to help us fight the battle and bring our thoughts back into line with what is right and pure.

There is no rest from this battle. We must *always* keep our guard up, because the moment we think, *It won't hit me here,* that is where it will hit us. The enemy is just waiting for us to relax and lower our defenses. So we need to consistently keep our armor on. Yet the Bible says we are not defenseless in this spiritual battle. We have been given powerful tools in this fight. Let's look at a key passage in Ephesians that illustrates this point.

Read Ephesians 6:10-19. Where does our strength lie (see v. 10)?

_____

_____

_____

What does this passage say we are struggling against (see v. 12)?

_____

_____

_____

Notice how many times these nine verses encourage us "to stand." What does it mean to "stand"?

_____

_____

_____

What are the specific pieces of armor we have available (see vv. 14-17)?

_____

_____

_____

What is our weapon in this battle (see v. 17)? How can that weapon help us to keep our thoughts in line with what is right and pure? (Hint: It's one of the reasons why you are encouraged to memorize the weekly Scripture verses!)

_____

_____

_____

In verse 18, Paul says to "pray in the Spirit on all occasions with all kinds of prayers and requests." How is this also a weapon in our fight?

_____

_____

_____

Notice in verse 19 that Paul indicates that he fights this spiritual battle because he is on a mission. What is his specific mission?

_____

_____

_____

What is your mission? How is being in a First Place 4 Health group a part of you fulfilling that mission?

_____

_____

_____

What have you learned in this lesson that will help you when you are struggling with your thoughts?

_____

_____

_____

Conclude today's study by doing as Paul suggests: go to God in prayer! Ask God to give you the strength to resist thinking on the things that are not from Him. Ask Him to give you the power to stand firm in the face of the enemy's attacks and resist his advances. For as James 4:7 says, "Submit yourselves . . . to God. Resist the devil, and he will flee from you."

Jesus, the battle belongs to You. I give You control over my mind, my thoughts, my heart and the behaviors that results. You are a righteous and magnificent God, and I purposefully remind myself of these truths. Amen.

A LOOK AT LOVELINESS

Jesus, help me always to focus my thoughts on You. I want to honor You today and every day with my thoughts, heart, words and deeds. Amen.

The word "loveliness" usually brings to mind physical beauty. But have you ever seen someone who may not necessarily be beautiful by the world's standards but is nonetheless a "lovely" person? This person is typically someone who has a spirit of graciousness, kindness or sweetness—one that comes from deep inside. Much the same way, if we look at the world around us through Christ's eyes, we will see what is truly lovely and worthy of our enjoyment. Things that are truly lovely inspire us. For instance, seeing a person lead a balanced life can be considered "lovely."

Today, we will look at a number of different verses to explore this idea of the word "lovely" and examine how focusing our minds on the things that are truly lovely is part of what it means to give Christ control over our lives.

"Lovely" means having qualities that inspire love or affection. The opposite is "repulsive." What does it look like when our thoughts are lovely?

_____

_____

_____

What does it look like when our thoughts are repulsive?

_____

_____

_____

Turn in your Bible to Psalm 84:1-2. How does the psalmist describe the dwelling place of God?

_____

_____

_____

How does he describe his response when he thinks about the dwelling place of the Lord and the living God?

_____

_____

_____

What is the dwelling place of God today? (See 1 Corinthians 6:19-20.)

_____

_____

_____

In what ways might the new dwelling place of God be considered lovely?

_____

_____

_____

"Pure" means being free from anything that taints, impairs or infects. What do 2 Corinthians 11:2 and 1 John 3:2-3 say about purity?

_____

_____

_____

What's the connection between giving Christ control over your mind and being pure of heart?

_____

_____

_____

What does Proverbs 15:26 say about the thoughts of the wicked in contrast to the thoughts of the pure?

_____

_____

_____

How does focusing on what is pure lead to true loveliness?

_____

_____

_____

Read Hebrews 2:18–3:1. How can these verses serve to encourage us?

_____

_____

_____

Jesus Himself suffered when He was tempted. He knows the struggles that we are going through, and He is able to help us. That should be a great encouragement to each of us!

Lord Jesus, You understand the struggles that I am going through. Today, help me to fix my mind on You and what You call good. Amen.

EXCELLENT AND PRAISEWORTHY

Day 5

Heavenly Father, You alone are worthy of my praise. Fill me with Your glory and bring my thoughts under your control. Amen.

A few years back, a book called _In Search of Excellence: Lessons from America's Best-Run Companies_ was released and quickly became a bestseller. In researching the material for the book, the authors searched for companies in America that operated with higher standards than others and were unwilling to compromise and settle for mediocrity. It made for quite an interesting premise—that excellence in business was so unusual that it attracted attention.[1]

What is excellent is worthy of praise. Ultimately, we live our lives in God's presence. His evaluation of us is the true measure of success. Whenever we allow mediocrity to fill our minds, we accept that which is second best. Our thoughts become distracted from God's standard.

The Bible consistently encourages us to set our standards high, beginning with the way we think.

Read Isaiah 6:1-8. How is the Lord described in this passage?

_____

_____

_____

What is Isaiah's response when he sees the Lord (see v. 5)?

_____

_____

_____

What is the seraph's response to Isaiah (see v. 7)? How is this same truth available in our lives today?

_____

_____

_____

Lamentations 3:23 states, "[The Lord's] compassions never fail. They are new every morning; great is your faithfulness." What does this verse tell us about the mercies of God? How might this verse apply to what's excellent (or not) in our thought life?

_____

_____

_____

"Excellent" means outstandingly good among its kind or of exceptional merit. "Praiseworthy" means commendable. Based on these definitions, what does it look like when our thoughts are excellent?

_____

_____

_____

In Psalm 8:1, David offers a praise to God, saying, "O Lord, our Lord, how majestic is your name in all the earth!" As you conclude today's study, spend a few moments focusing on the excellence of God and how He has revealed His majesty in your life. He is worthy of our praise!

Lord Jesus, by Your grace I am made excellent, inside and out. I rely on this grace in my life. Help me always to focus on what is excellent. Amen.

REFLECTION AND APPLICATION

Day
6

God, You are the epitome of whatever is true, noble, right, pure, lovely, excellent and praiseworthy. Today, I invite You to fill me with these qualities.

An excellent way to keep our thoughts centered on good things is to fill our minds with God's Word. Having Scripture in our hearts and minds helps us focus on those things that lead us to worship God. It's much harder for the evil one to get a foothold in our lives when our minds are filled with Scripture. Scripture and right thinking crowd the evil one out, leaving room only for God. Strongholds cannot stand against the Word of God.

Today, simply spend some time in prayer. Ask God to help you think what is right and pleasing to Him. If you prefer, you can use some of the prayers given below.

God, may the words of my mouth and meditations of my heart be pleasing in Your sight, for You are my Rock and my Redeemer (see Psalm 19:14).

O Lord, I know You that have searched me and know me when I sit or when I rise. You perceive my thoughts from afar. Please help me to keep my thoughts focused on You. Fill me with Your Holy Spirit (see Psalm 139:1-2).

Search me, O God, and know my heart; test me and know my anxious thoughts. See if there is any offensive way in me, and lead me in the way everlasting (see Psalm 139:23-24).

REFLECTION AND APPLICATION

*Oh Lord, help me always keep my mind on You and what
is pleasing to You. You are good. You are loving. You care for me.
I love You. Amen.*

In her book *Praying God's Word*, Beth Moore says that churches tend to give the devil either too much credit or not nearly enough. She also states that Satan has successfully duped the vast majority of churches into an imbalance as it relates to all things concerning or threatening him.[2]

Our sure defense against evil is to be steeped in the Word of God. Sin crouches at our doors just waiting to devour us (see Genesis 4:7), so we must continually be armed for the battle that rages all around us. Whenever we pursue the heart of Christ and all things concerning Him, we win this battle.

The invitation today is for you to think about Christ and what is pleasing to Him. To help give your mind some mental pictures, in the spaces below write down some things that will help you to continually fix your mind on Christ.

When I think of Christ's beauty, I picture . . .

_____

_____

_____

When I think of Christ's majesty, I picture . . .

_____

_____

_____

When I think of whatever is true and noble, I picture . . .

_____

_____

_____

When I think of whatever is righteous and pure, I picture . . .

_____

_____

_____

When I think of whatever is admirable and excellent, I picture . . .

_____

_____

_____

Whenever I think of whatever is lovely, I picture . . .

_____

_____

_____

> *Lord, thank You for adopting me into Your family. Thank You for Your glorious grace, which You have freely given to me through Christ Jesus (see Ephesians 1:4-6). Today, I will yield to Your glory and focus on whatever is noble, pure, lovely, admirable, excellent and praiseworthy.*

Notes
1. Thomas J. Peters and Robert H. Waterman, *In Search of Excellence: Lessons from America's Best-Run Companies* (New York: Warner Books, 1982).
2. Beth Moore, *Praying God's Word* (Nashville, TN: Broadman and Holman Publishers, 2000), p. 309.

Group Prayer Requests

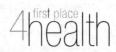

Today's Date: _____

Name	Request

Results

_____

_____

_____

_____

_____

control: whose responsibility is it?

SCRIPTURE MEMORY VERSE

I have been crucified with Christ and I no longer live, but Christ lives in me. The life I live in the body, I live by faith in the Son of God, who loved me and gave himself for me.

GALATIANS 2:20

Giving Christ control over our lives does not mean that we lack self-control. It actually a bit of a paradox: We are always responsible for our actions, yet we relinquish ultimate control to the Lord. Self-control and being controlled by Christ always go hand in hand.

It is necessary for us to understand that we are always invited to live self-controlled lives, because when life slips out of control, it's often convenient for us to want to pass the buck—to shift the blame to other people or situations. We might say things such as:

"He made me do it."
"The temptation was too strong."
"It caught me at a weak moment."
"I didn't think it could happen to me."
"I deserved to have this one lapse in judgment."

This week, we will look at God's invitation to us to always lead lives that are self-controlled. We will see how God equips us to be responsible for our actions while, at the same time, giving control to Him and resting in His provision.

Day
1

SHIFTING THE BLAME

Lord, You created me with a will. My life is in Your hands, and You respect me so much that You are willing to give me decision-making power. Amen.

Since the very beginning of the Bible, people have struggled with self-control. The book of Genesis tells how the first two people responded after they lost control of their lives. Today, we will take a look at this story a bit more closely.

Before we begin, however, we first need to take a look at our own lives. Given the opportunity, it's easy for us to shift the blame when we are confronted with mistakes, sin or out-of-balance situations. When our lives seem out of balance, who (or what) do we generally look to as being responsible for the problem? Ourselves? God? Our boss? Our spouse? Our kids? Our parents?

Think about a recent experience you faced in which you realized that things were out of balance. How did you respond to that situation?

_____

_____

_____

Now turn in your Bible to Genesis 3:8-13. As we pick up the story, Adam and Eve have just eaten from the Tree of the Knowledge of Good and Evil in violation of God's command. How did they first react when they heard the sound of the Lord walking in the Garden (see v. 8)?

_____

_____

_____

How did God know that they had disobeyed His command (see v. 11)?

_____

_____

_____

God then asks Adam and Eve to explain their actions. How did Adam respond (see v. 12)?

_____

_____

_____

_____

God created us in His image and gave us the freedom to make moral choices, and He holds us responsible for those choices we make. Scripture indicates that shifting blame is not an option; we are accountable to God for our actions. Of course, the ultimate decision for which we are all responsible is whether we decide to accept or reject Christ's offer of salvation. God works in the hearts of all people, drawing them to seek and receive Christ, and only in Christ is the powerful grip of sin broken. Once we become Christians, we die to sin's domination and Christ takes up residence in our lives. Through His powerful life in us, He enables us to resist and overcome the desire to sin.

Look up Romans 6:2 and Galatians 5:24. What common idea is presented in these verses? What does this look like in everyday life?

_____

_____

_____

_____

Once we were slaves to sin. We were controlled and dominated, and only through death could we find release. But because of Christ's death and resurrection for us, we have the option of being liberated from our sin. Spiritually speaking, we are invited to die and live again through Christ. Look up Romans 6:11. What does this verse say about sin and death?

_____

_____

_____

Because sin can no longer dominate our lives when we become Christians, what force now controls our lives?

_____

_____

_____

_____

Once we accept Christ, the Holy Spirit is now free to work in our lives and help us control the temptations that come our way. How have you seen this work in action in your own life? (Think about some of the struggles you faced that led you to joining First Place 4 Health and how God has helped you to overcome.)

_____

_____

_____

In what ways do you want the Holy Spirit to take control?

_____

_____

_____

In Matthew 12:29, Jesus asks, "How can anyone enter a strong man's house and carry off his possessions unless he first ties up the strong man? Then he can rob his house." If you have entrusted your life to Christ as your Savior, He has entered in and bound up the "strong man." You are no longer in bondage to your past. You have been set free from the suffocating control of sin. So, as you conclude today's study, take some time to pray right now and thank God for His gift of salvation.

Oh Lord, thank You for freeing me from the control of sin. I yield my life to You. Help me to always walk in Your pathways. Amen.

A STRATEGY FOR FIGHTING TEMPTATION

Thank You, Father, for providing what I need when my life spins out of control. Please give me the strength I need to follow You. Amen.

What should we do when harmful thoughts roll around in our heads and prompt us to move toward sinful actions? In these matters, we always have a choice. Scripturally, we know that sin has no authority in our lives as believers. Temptation is not an irresistible influence. We are free! When we are tempted, we need to remind ourselves that we no longer have to respond to sin's demands. We are dead to sin, and it no longer reigns in our lives.

However, in spite of everything God has done to empower us to not sin, sometimes we still find ourselves succumbing to temptation. Fortunately, God always provides a way out, even when life slips out of balance. The Bible acknowledges that people will still sin, even after they become Christians.

Turn to 1 John 1:9-10. What remedy for sin is offered in verse 9?

_____

_____

_____

What does the author say in verse 10 about the need for us to be honest with our personal failings? Rewrite this passage in your own words.

_____

_____

_____

When faced with temptation, God invites us to yield our hearts to Him and bring our actions back on track. The foundation for our authority to do this is found in Romans 6:11-13. Now, although the principles in this passage might sound somewhat abstract at first, they lay a solid foundation of spiritual truth from which we can operate.

Read Romans 6:11-13. What is the first principle Paul explains in verse 11?

_____

_____

_____

What is the second principle he explains in verse 12?

_____

_____

_____

What do we need to offer to God in verse 13—the third principle?

_____

_____

_____

Let's make these ideas really practical. Imagine a situation in which your heart and actions are tempted in a manner that goes against God's plan for righteousness. How can you apply the three principles of Romans 6:11-13 to choose heart responses and actions that please God?

I count myself dead to sin by . . .

_____

_____

_____

I don't let sin reign in my life by . . .

_____

_____

_____

I offer every part of my life to God by . . .

_____

_____

_____

Conclude today's session by taking a good look at any area of your life where you have not followed these principles. Confess these to God, and then rest in the assurance that He is gracious and just to free you from all unrighteousness.

Lord, thank You for freeing me from sin's control. Thank You
for the victory You have provided through the death of Your Son
on the cross. I yield my life to You today and every day. Amen.

PRINCIPLES FOR LIVING A GODLY LIFE

Day
3

Jesus, You endured the cross to set me free from sin so I could have access to
the Father. Holy Spirit, You fill my life, transforming me into the image of
the Son, giving me new power each day. I love You. Amen.

Even armed with spiritual truth, situations can develop that push us to the limits. At times, the attraction of sin and enticement of temptation can feel too powerful to resist. But any time we give in to temptation, our lives spin out of control. Sin always hurts us, as well as the people we love. So today, we will examine a few additional principles in 1 Corinthians 10:1-13 to help us fight the war—principles that we need to know and ingest in order to resist temptation.

Paul begins this passage by offering some warnings from Israel's history. What are some of the examples he gives about how God had provided for them in their journey to the Promised Land (see vv. 1-4)?

_____

_____

_____

The Israelites witnessed the power of God. By day He guided them in a pillar of cloud, and at night by a pillar of fire (see Exodus 13:21). He led them safely through the sea when they were fleeing the Egyptians (see Exodus 14:16-17). He gave them manna to eat in the desert (see Exodus

16:4) and water from a stone (see Exodus 17:5-6). Nevertheless, Paul says that God was not pleased with them. What was the reason for this (see 1 Corinthians 10:6)?

_____

_____

_____

What examples does Paul give of the ways that the Israelites "set [their] hearts on evil things" (see vv. 7-10)?

_____

_____

_____

What is the reason Paul gives for why these stories were recorded in the Bible (see v. 11)?

_____

_____

_____

In verse 13, Paul provides an explanation of the five principles we need to know and to resist temptation. Study the verse, and then fill in the chart below.

Principle	What this principle might look like in my life
Temptation is common	
God is faithful	
The limits of temptation have been set	

Principle	What this principle might look like in my life
There's always a way out	
We can stand firm under pressure	

Lord, help me to always think through a strategy to avoid temptation.
Help me to be prepared to fight the attacks of the enemy when they come.
I want to follow these principles when temptation comes my way so that
I can serve You with my whole life. You are a glorious God. Amen.

POWER IN WEAKNESS

Day 4

Thank You, Father, for providing a way for temptation
to never overpower my life. I praise You for providing a way
for me to escape the snares of the enemy. Amen.

In the process of giving Christ control over our lives, there may be times when we feel weak. Sin's unrelenting assault against us can create spiritual pressure, even exhaustion. In desperation, we may cry out for help and strength. But during such times, we can rest assured that help is available. The Lord promises to help us in our times of need. We will take a closer look at this today.

What's the true motivation for giving Christ control of our lives? Is it simply to avoid negative consequences from sinning, or is there something more? (Hint: see Colossians 1:10 and Ephesians 4:1.)

_____

_____

_____

Read 2 Corinthians 12:8-10. What is happening to Paul here?

_____

_____

_____

What is his prayer to the Lord?

_____

_____

_____

What is God's answer to Paul?

_____

_____

_____

What is Paul's conclusion about God's answer?

_____

_____

_____

God hears us when we cry out to Him. Whenever we are weak, He gives us strength. He uses the weakest areas of our life as a platform to exhibit His power. He promises never to leave us or forsake us. The following verses reveal principles about God's power in our lives. Read each passage, then write the central idea of the Scripture as it relates to your life.

Passage	Central idea as it relates to your life
Romans 4:20-21	
Ephesians 3:16-21	

Passage	Central idea as it relates to your life
Ephesians 6:10	
2 Timothy 1:17	
Colossians 1:29	
2 Peter 1:3	

God has the power to overcome any difficulty we might face. He has the power to do what He has promised. In what area of your life do you need the presence of God today? Spend a few minutes and take these issues to the Lord in prayer.

Lord, thank You for giving me strength to face the struggles that threaten to overcome me. I give these to You today and rely on Your strength. Amen.

THE WISDOM OF BOUNDARIES

Day 5

Thank you Father for providing a way for temptation to never overpower my life. I praise You for providing a way for me to escape the snares of temptation. Help lead me to greater victory over sin. Amen.

Christians sometimes find themselves in difficult situations, particularly when they minister in the public arena. Billy Graham once said, "My greatest fear is that I'll do something or say something that will bring disrepute on the gospel of Christ." Graham was always reported to be cautious in guarding himself against sexual sin. For instance, he made it a policy that neither he nor any other male member of his staff was every permitted to be in a room alone with a female (who wasn't the man's spouse) unless the door was kept open. Similarly, Graham never opened a hotel room until an aide had first checked it. Was he paranoid? No, he was simply realistic about the power of sin and the battle that Christians must wage to resist its pull.

Read 1 Corinthians 8:1-11. In this passage, Paul was dealing with a specific problem in the church in Corinth: whether believers should eat food sacrificed to idols. What does he say about idols in verse 4?

_____

_____

_____

What does he say about the one Lord we serve in verses 5-6? Where does Paul stands on this issue based on these verses?

_____

_____

_____

However, Paul adds a caveat in verse 7. What does he see as the problem with Christians eating food sacrificed to idols?

_____

_____

_____

Notice in verse 9 that Paul states, "Be careful, however, that the exercise of your freedom does not become a stumbling block to the weak." How can a careless action on your part have a negative impact on another person? (Make this example specific to your life and your participation in First Place 4 Health.)

_____

_____

_____

According to Paul, what is the danger in you setting such an example for another believer (see vv. 10-11)?

_____

_____

_____

One powerful way for us to overcome sin is to establish boundaries before we are tempted to sin. Then, when temptation strikes, we don't need to rely solely on our willpower. Willpower by itself is weak, but willpower combined with the strength of the Holy Spirit is powerful.

One of the tools the Holy Spirit provides is prudence. The Holy Spirit invites us to use prudence to set up healthy boundaries so we can live freely and safely within those boundaries. Think of prudence as the wisdom to act rationally, sensibly, logically and wisely in real life.

As you conclude today's study, take some time to think about your greatest temptations. Then think of a few ways that you can set up healthy boundaries before these temptations strike. As you do this, remember that boundaries aren't just for actions: Christ is equally concerned about the attitude of your heart as well.

Heavenly Father, thank You for Your wisdom. Help me to set up appropriate boundaries in my life. I want to follow You with all my heart. Amen.

REFLECTION AND APPLICATION

Day 6

Thank You, God, for giving me resources to overcome temptation so I can glorify You and lead a healthy life. Amen.

This week, we have studied about our responsibility in choosing to avoid evil. We looked at how Christ gives us power as we make right choices and how it's our responsibility to work with Him to overcome temptation. Christ always invites us to work in partnership with Him. He is ultimately in control, yet He invites us to be willful participants in the process.

One additional God-given resource we have in this area is accountability. Accountability simply means that others walk this journey with us and help us set a healthy course and stay on track. An accountability partner could be a trusted friend or mentor that we check in with at certain points during the week to discuss any issues we may be facing. He or she can serve a voice of wisdom in our lives and give us practical advice for how to overcome certain struggles. God can use these individuals to strengthen us and provide the support we need during difficult times. And we can provide the same to them.

Take some time today to contact a trusted friend—by phone, email or letter, or perhaps you can even meet for coffee or lunch—and spend some time talking through the things that you have learned this week.

Thank You God, for giving me resources to help me live a life that pleases You. Thank You for continually leading me in the way everlasting. Amen.

Day 7 REFLECTION AND APPLICATION

Lord, help me to always keep my mind on You and what is pleasing to You. Thank You for giving me an abundant life. You are good. You are loving. You care for me. I love You. Amen.

In John 10:10, Jesus said, "The thief comes only to steal and kill and destroy; I have come that they may have life, and have it to the full." A stronghold is any familiar sin that causes us to stumble and give in to temptation. It's anything that steals, kills, or destroys the abundant life we have in Christ.

God is more powerful than any stronghold we may have. Whether that stronghold involves poor eating habits, harmful relationships with others, a rebellious spirit, pride or feelings of guilt, God can overcome it. He sent the Holy Spirit to give us power so that we can break our strongholds and be set free!

God equips us with His Word, prayer, accountability and the prudence to set healthy boundaries. He does this to help us overcome any sinful habits or desires we may have. He wants to change us so that we intrinsically want to pursue heart attitudes and actions that are healthy. He wants to build us up so that we also can encourage those around us and ultimately glorify Him. God's desire for us is to be successful in all our endeavors that are in accordance to His will for our lives.

Today, take a few minutes to look up the following verses in your Bible and then spend some time meditating on the truth contained in each passage. Read through each verse prayerfully. You may also want to journal about what the Lord has been teaching you lately.

Psalm 26:2-3

_____

_____

_____

Psalm 86:11

_____

_____

_____

John 15:26

_____

_____

_____

Galatians 2:20

_____

_____

_____

Heavenly Father, You are more powerful than any stronghold in my life. Thank You for giving me the power to break free from the things that have bound me in the past. I give the control to You. Amen.

Group Prayer Requests

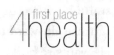

Today's Date: _____

Name	Request

Results

_____

_____

_____

_____

_____

yielding our desires

SCRIPTURE MEMORY VERSE
*I have learned the secret of being content in any and every situation,
whether well fed or hungry, whether living in plenty or in want.
I can do everything through him who gives me strength.*
PHILIPPIANS 4:12-13

Several years ago, a cartoon in a newspaper pictured two mules standing in adjoining pastures of lush green grass separated by a tightly strung barbed-wire fence. Each mule had poked his head through the fence and was attempting to eat the grass in the next pasture while pressing against the barbs. Under the image, the cartoonist had written one word: "Discontent."

"Discontent" could be defined as the restless desire for something more or different. It is the condition of feeling displeased or dissatisfied with something in life. Of course, it's not always wrong to be discontented. In fact, sometimes Christ instills in us a godly discontent that presses us to do His will or pushes us forward into greater health and wholeness. But often, discontent can be birthed out of ungratefulness or the wrong type of ambition. In a world driven by this type of discontentedness, God offers the only antidote: letting Him take the wheel of our lives.

In this week's study, we will examine three negative emotions that fuel this harmful type of discontent: lust, greed and envy. We will examine the opposite of this—spiritual contentment—and how to develop that quality in our lives.

TRUE CONTENTMENT

*God, You created me with a will. I have the power to choose whether to go
right or left, up or down. Help me to choose the path of contentment. Amen.*

Desire fuels discontent, which may channel itself through lust, greed and
envy. Once any of these emotions begins to surge through us, our lives
can readily skid out of control. The power of these negative emotions can
cause us to struggle even more as we try to resist temptation and please
God. For these reasons we cannot allow these emotions to reside unchal-
lenged in our lives, for once entrenched, they tend to wreak havoc.

It's been said that contentment is when a person thinks about yesterday without regret and tomorrow without fear. That's a pretty close
definition. Actually, true contentment occurs when we place our lives
fully in God's hands. Sure, we are still responsible for our own choices
and actions, but we've yielded both our ultimate destiny and our day-to-
day destinies to the Lord. Who we meet, the jobs we get, the person we
marry, the children we have, the breaks we get or don't get, where we live,
what happens to us—all of this is ultimately up to God.

God allows us to have choices, but all our lives are ultimately under
His reign. We learn to rest easy when we know that everything that happens to us and for us passes first through the filter of His good and
righteous character and is within His permissive will.

Begin today's study by reading Philippians 4:10-13. What was the occa-
sion for Paul's rejoicing in verse 10?

_____

_____

_____

The context of why Paul was expressing his great joy actually appears a
few verses later in this passage. At the time that Paul was writing this
letter, he was in prison. A messenger had arrived from the church in
Philippi with gifts for him (see v. 18). Paul was grateful not just for the

gifts but also for what it represented: evidence of that church renewing their concern for him. Yet Paul is quick to add a disclaimer in verse 11. What does he state about his contentment in that verse?

_____

_____

_____

_____

What does Paul say he has learned through his experience in verse 12?

_____

_____

_____

What was Paul's secret of "being content in any and every situation"?

_____

_____

_____

Turn to 1 Timothy 6:6. What is Paul saying about true contentment in this verse?

_____

_____

_____

In Hebrews 13:5, we read, "Keep your lives free from the love of money and be content with what you have, because God has said, 'Never will I leave you; never will I forsake you.'" What attitude does the writer of Hebrews exhort us to adopt as it relates to seeking contentment in the things of this world?

_____

_____

_____

What leads to true contentment, according this verse?

_____

_____

_____

It is possible to be content regardless of the circumstances we experience. Paul faced incredible obstacles in his life, far more than most Christians typically encounter. Yet in each situation, he tested one simple idea: *If I have Christ, will I have all I need?* Over and over again, whether in want or in plenty, Paul found that Christ's grace was sufficient, and His power was made perfect in weakness. As you conclude today's study, read Psalm 37:7 and Psalm 46:10. Spend some time praying through these verses, asking the Lord to help you be content in all circumstances.

> *Lord, You are over all, and in all, and through all. You are Lord over everything. All the earth is in Your hands. I rest in that knowledge. Amen.*

Day 2 LUST: DESIRES OUT OF CONTROL

Dear God, help me always to want only what You want. Amen.

God wants the desires of our hearts to be closely connected with His. That's one of the foundational principles upon which First Place 4 Health is based. In Matthew 6:33, Jesus encourages us to seek first His kingdom and His righteousness. When we do that—when what we seek is aligned with God's desires—the rest of our lives follow suit and fall into place. We live as we were truly meant to live.

Desires that are out of control fall under the category of "lust." Lust means that we want to gratify our senses or appetites with no thought as to the outcome. For instance, if we lust for food, we aren't giving thought to the results or repercussions of what we are putting into our bodies—our only aim is to quench our thirst or satiate our appetite or, typically, fill an empty spot in our souls. Whenever we lust, we will not experience the joy of contentment.

Turn to Ephesians 4:17-24. As you read this passage, keep in mind that Paul is writing to Gentiles (those of non-Jewish heritage) who have converted to the Christian faith. What does Paul say that these individuals must not do in verses 17-19?

_____

_____

_____

_____

Paul then reminds these believers that they certainly did not come to know Christ by having such a "darkened" understanding of the Christian life. What does he remind them they were taught when they decided to follow Christ (see v. 22)?

_____

_____

_____

_____

What does Paul tell them that the attitudes of their minds should be (see vv. 23-24)?

_____

_____

_____

_____

In 1 Timothy 6:11, Paul writes, "But you, man of God, flee from all this, and pursue righteousness, godliness, faith, love, endurance and gentleness." When it comes to lust, what is Paul's practical advice for Timothy—and for us?

_____

_____

_____

_____

What practical advice for avoiding lust do we find in Psalm 25:15?

_____

_____

_____

What are some ways we can continually keep our eyes on the Lord?

_____

_____

_____

Read Psalm 105:4 and Isaiah 55:1-3. What does God offer as an antidote to lust?

_____

_____

_____

Oh Lord, all goodness and joy is found in You. You are the provider by Your sufficient grace. Help me to know this truth and to live by it. Amen.

Day 3

GREED: WHEN WE CONTINUALLY WANT MORE

Dear God, again I will pray this simple prayer: Help me always to want only what You want. Amen.

If you ever travel to India, South Africa or Saudi Arabia, there is something you must be wary of: monkeys.[1] Aggressive monkeys have become quite a problem in some of the tourist areas of these countries. The problem is that they are greedy. If you have a bunch of bananas and offer one to a monkey, he will typically ignore it and try to grab the entire bunch. If you hand out something that they don't typically eat, like sugar cookies, peanuts or Pop Tarts, they will fight among themselves over it. If you've got something they want, they have no problem biting, slapping or shoving you to get it.

Greed is something we want that's beyond us, that we want with an unmatched intensity, and that we want without thought as to how we get it or whom it might harm. It's a self-serving desire for money, wealth, power, food or other possessions, especially when this denies the same goods to others. It's like the monkey who is not content with the single banana offered to him and instead goes for the entire bunch—without regard to the person holding it. The Bible describes greed as one of the all-encompassing sins we must continually battle. Contentment will continue to elude us as long as greed undercuts our satisfaction.

Let's look at a few passages today on how we can prevent greed in our lives.

In Luke 12:13-21, Jesus tells the parable of the rich fool. What was the situation that prompted Jesus to tell this parable (see vv. 13-14)?

_____

_____

_____

_____

The Jewish laws at the time covered most of the provisions about who inherited what when someone died, but sometimes there was room for doubt. In this case, the man felt that his brother was doing an injustice to him, and he wanted Jesus to intervene. The man was treating Jesus as a typical rabbi, who customarily gave decisions on disputed points of law. But how does Jesus respond (see v. 14)?

_____

_____

_____

What does He specifically say about greed in verse 15?

_____

_____

_____

Jesus then begins to tell the parable. What is the problem that the rich man has? What is his solution (see vv. 16-19)?

_____

_____

_____

It's not wrong for people to save, invest and expand their business if they have been blessed. What was wrong with the rich man's motives in choosing to tear down his barns to build more?

_____

_____

God wants us to use the resources He has given to us wisely, and He wants us to bless others with those resources. The man in this parable is not interested in helping others with wealth. He's not even that interested in making a fuller life for himself. He is concerned solely with self-indulgence. What does God say about this man's attitude (see v. 20)?

_____

_____

_____

What point was Jesus making to the man who had the dispute over his inheritance with his brother?

_____

_____

_____

Read Exodus 20:17 and Romans 7:7-8. How seriously does God take the problem of greed, or wanting something so badly that you covet it?

_____

_____

_____

Paul also had to confront greed in the Early Church. In Ephesians 5:5, he writes, "No immoral, impure or greedy person—such a man is an idolater—has any inheritance in the kingdom of Christ and of God." How does Paul classify a greedy person? What is his stern warning to him or her in this verse?

_____

_____

_____

According to Hosea 10:12, what is the remedy to greed?

_____

_____

_____

Lord, grant me contentment and satisfaction in this life based on my relationship with You. Help me keep my eyes focused only on You. Amen.

ENVY: MAKING COMPARISIONS

Day 4

Dear God, help me not to compare myself against any false standard of success. Help me to focus solely on You and Your will for my life. Amen.

The Roman philosopher Lucius Annaeus Seneca (5 BC–AD 65) once said, "Not he who has little, but he who wishes for more is poor." Lust seeks selfish gratification of the senses. Greed wants more but is never satisfied. Envy disparages others for perceived advantages.

When we are "envious," it means that we feel discontent and ill will because of another person's success. It's a feeling of resentment that comes when someone has something that we want. And because the focus of envy is on other people having things we don't have, it is not unusual that others are hurt, directly or indirectly, as a result of our envy. At the very least, it strains our relationship (or potential relationship) with them.

Are you guilty of being envious? Here's a short test. Have you ever said anything to yourself such as:

- Why is that person so thin? I exercise a lot more.
- Why do they have such a nice house? It seems like everyone has a nice place to live except us.
- Why is that person so talented? She seems to be good at everything. It's not fair.
- Why does she catch all the breaks? I've been working forever and getting nowhere.

Have you ever felt this way? If so, you may need to get rid of envy in your life. Today, we will study a passage in James that shows us how.

Read James 3:13-4:6. According to James, what is the source of envy (see vv. 14-15)?

_____

_____

_____

What are the harmful results that envy produces (see v. 16)?

_____

_____

_____

How does one get the type of wisdom shown in verses 17-18?

_____

_____

_____

In James 4:1-3, the author describes greed in all its ugliness. How does he then say that humility is an antidote to envy (see vv. 4-6)?

_____

_____

_____

What is another antidote to envy as shown in Philippians 4:19?

_____

_____

_____

Conclude today's study by taking a good look at this issue in your life. Have you been envious of others? If so, look to God and rest in Him, knowing that He will meet all of your needs. Concentrate on the fact that He has a particular plan for *your* life—and that plan doesn't involve what others might have that you don't!

Lord, help me always to approach You with a sincere heart and a clean conscious, desiring only what You want for me. Amen.

RELEASING THE HOSTAGES

Day 5

Dear God, I come before You as a sinner saved by grace. Help me not to lust, be greedy or to envy others. I yield these areas of my life to You. Help me, Lord, for I am in need. Amen.

Because we have been given new life in Christ, there is nothing that can hold us as spiritual hostages. We are free from sin. Christ has given us the power we need to have the victory over these negative pulls in our lives. Yet the emotional drives of lust, greed and envy continually tend to be strong and destructive. Sometimes, it's hard to believe that we are truly free.

In today's study, we will look at a passage of Scripture in Matthew 19:16-22. In this story, Jesus meets a rich young man who wants to know what he needs to do to obtain eternal life. As you read this passage, it is important to note that in culture of the time, it was often assumed that wealth was a sign of God's blessing. Most religious teachers would be assumed to have at least some wealth. This made Jesus and His disciples stand out.

What was the man's question? How did Jesus respond (see vv. 16-17)?

_____

_____

_____

Based on the young man's response in verse 20, was he a "good" person?

_____

_____

_____

The young man realized that although he had kept these commandments, he still lacked something. What did Jesus say that he had to do to be "perfect" (see v. 21)?

_____

_____

_____

What was the young man's response (see v. 22)?

_____

_____

_____

Jesus viewed the rich young man's attitude as a form of greed. He had become a slave to his possessions. He had chosen to remain a spiritual hostage because he wasn't willing to give up all that he had to go and follow God. If the man had remained and spoken with Jesus some more, how do you think their conversation would have continued? Write some ideas below.

_____

_____

_____

_____

Now, we know from Scripture that there were those among Jesus' followers who had at least *some* money. In fact, He and His companions seemed to have depended upon some of these patrons for support (see Luke 8:3). The issue here was one of the heart: the rich young man was unwilling to give up that which mattered the most to him. What did Jesus say in Matthew 6:24 that illustrates this point?

_____

_____

_____

So, whom do you serve? Are you experiencing the freedom that Christ brings, or are you still struggling with an area of temptation? Have you surrendered that area of your life to God and experienced His mercy? If not, why not stop right now and simply ask the Lord to help you overcome an area of temptation. Invite the power of the Holy Spirit to come into your life and change your thinking. Remember that you can learn to be content in every situation because you can do everything through Christ Jesus who gives you strength. He will provide you with strength you need to do anything He has required.

Thank You, Father God, for helping me continue to conquer the negative influences of lust, greed and envy in my life. Please continue to teach me how You can fully satisfy the needs of my life. I surrender all to You. Amen.

REFLECTION AND APPLICATION

Day 6

Thank You, God, for giving me the resources to overcome temptation. I want to glorify You and live a balanced and healthy life. Amen.

This week, we studied how greed, lust and envy can sneak into our lives and cause imbalance, pain and chaos. Continually, we're invited in Scripture to turn away from negative emotions and steer toward God by the power of His Holy Spirit. One way to do this is to read His Word and memorize Scripture. But first, let's take a personal inventory. Of the various issues we've talked about this week, which, if any, would you say you struggle with the most? (Feel free to write the answer below or in your prayer journal.)

_____

_____

_____

The Bible provides us with great insight and ideas that can help us yield control to Christ. In the chart below, look up each of the Scripture verses. Write a short principle based on that verse in the right-hand column as it relates to how to overcome lust, greed or envy.

Emotion	Principle I can use to overcome the emotion
Lust	2 Timothy 2:22: Titus 2:11-12: 1 Peter 4:2:
Greed	Luke 12:15: Ephesians 5:3: 1 Peter 5:2:
Envy	1 Corinthians 13:4: Galatians 5:25-26: 1 Peter 2:1-2:

Holy Father, Your Word says that everything in the world—the cravings of my sinful nature, the lust of my eyes and the boasting of what I have and do—comes not from You but from the world and my flesh. You promised that the world and its desires will pass away, but the one who does Your will lives forever. Help me to live in Your will today (see 1 John 2:16-17). Amen.

REFLECTION AND APPLICATION

Day 7

Lord, thank You for the blessings in my life. Help me to continually yield my life to You. I love You, Lord. I want to follow You all my days. Amen.

Prayer is so important, so today we will spend some more time in prayer. Again, we will use the words of Scripture to guide us. God's Word is perfect, and the Bible verses we will memorize throughout this study and elsewhere will become the landmarks for seeking God's will and plan for our lives. Memorizing verses can serve as a beacon of light to help guide us during times of stress, temptation or difficulty.

As you conclude this week's study, remember the different weapons you can employ to fight lust, greed, envy and other temptations that come your way. You have the power of the Holy Spirit to help you in your time of need. You have the Word of God that you can hide in your heart to refute the advances of the enemy. You have the fellowship of other believers to help keep you accountable. You also have the power of prayer. Let's do that right now.

Lord, Your Word is clear that those who are self-seeking and who reject the truth and follow evil will experience Your wrath and anger. I don't want that. Help me to seek Your face always (see Romans 2:8).

Father God, continue to teach me. Help me to recognize what is in accordance with the truth that is in Jesus (see Ephesians 4:21).

Lord, thank You for the grace, mercy and peace that come from You and from Your Son, Jesus Christ, who is with me in truth and love (see 2 John 3).

Lord, help me to learn the secret of being content in any and every situation, whether I am well-fed or hungry, living in plenty or in want. I can do everything through You who gives me strength (see Philippians 4:12-13). Amen.

Note
1. Yes, there are monkeys in Saudi Arabia. In 2007, an aggressive pack of baboons took over an abandoned building in the capital of Riyadh and launched a raid on the city's outdoor markets.

Group Prayer Requests

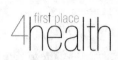

Today's Date: _____

Name	Request

Results

_____

_____

_____

_____

_____

releasing
our calling

SCRIPTURE MEMORY VERSE
*Do not think of yourself more highly than you ought,
but rather think of yourself with sober judgment,
in accordance with the measure of faith God has given you.*
ROMANS 12:3

In her memoir *Angels of a Lower Flight*, Susan Scott Krabacher describes how she spent two decades of her youth wrongly focused inward on herself. She writes, "My ambition had been to transform myself into someone who would be loved. Not satisfied with my natural state, I spent days at the hair salon and gym, manicuring, pedicuring, soaking, dyeing, running, tanning, waxing and dieting."[1]

Susan falsely believed that her life was completely in her hands, so she clutched and clawed her way to some of the highest rungs of the modeling industry. At one point she had everything—money, fame, big houses, fancy cars, the love of a powerful man. But inside she was empty and desperate. Her life soon crashed down around her.

From the bottom, she allowed the Lord to remake her life. She yielded control of her life to God and discovered that everything that had happened to her had happened for a purpose. The Lord led her to a new career as cofounder and CEO of the Mercy and Sharing Foundation, a humanitarian organization that ministers among the world's poorest of the poor in Haiti. Although the work is seldom easy, Susan has never been more content.

God may not make the same radical call on all of our lives as He did for Susan Krabacher's, but the same principles hold true. We can clutch and claw at our lives, hoping to control the success and purpose that comes to us, or we can release our lives and our future into God's hands.

Day 1 — RELEASING OUR RÉSUMÉS

O gracious God, I invite You to fully guide my life. You know more about me than I do about myself. I release my future into Your hands. Amen.

It's easy to want to control our futures. Many of us spend a great deal of time, energy and effort "inventing" ourselves. We strive to create a look, image and résumé that will garner the right sort of attention, perhaps propelling us into the right position or leading us to what we hope will be the perfect location. But what happens when that perfectly crafted résumé gets off track from what we'd hoped?

The patriarch Joseph began his life with a perfect résumé. He was the favored son of Isaac, a prominent tribal leader. As a young man, Joseph had much to look forward to. He was given a coat of many colors, a symbol of honor and privilege, and he began having dreams and visions. It looked as if God was smiling in a special way on this young man. But very soon, situations beyond Joseph's control began to change all that.

Read Genesis 37:1-10. In his youthful exuberance, what things does Joseph do that could be described as mistakes (see vv. 6-7)?

_____

_____

_____

Read Genesis 37:23-28 and 39:6-20. By the time Joseph is a young man, probably not yet 20 years old, what two "blotches" are on his résumé?

_____

_____

_____

Read Genesis 39:21-22. Even when Joseph is in the lowest places in his life, what wonderful spiritual truth is also evident in his life?

_____

_____

_____

In what ways have you seen God's presence in your life, even at your lowest times?

_____

_____

_____

If you are familiar with the story of Joseph, you know that while he is in prison, he correctly interprets the dreams of two of Pharaoh's officials (see Genesis 40–41). Later, when Pharaoh needs a dream interpreted, one of Pharaoh's officials (who has since been released from prison) remembers Joseph. Joseph correctly interprets Pharaoh's dream, is released from prison, and is appointed second-in-command of all of Egypt. What do you think Joseph might have learned from all his years of waiting on the Lord?

_____

_____

_____

_____

Much later, Joseph describes how the events of his life have been brought together for a purpose. Read Genesis 45:4-8. What similar confidence do we have? How have you seen evidence of this in your own life or in people you've known?

_____

_____

_____

_____

Lord, let my dreams be Your dreams, my ambitions Your ambitions, and my goals Your goals. Let me want nothing other than Your plan for my life.

Day 2 · RELEASING OUR DESTINATIONS

Lord, where do You want me to be? What plans do You have for my family and loved ones? Let me be in the places and situations that You ordain. Amen.

Have you ever longed to live in a particular location, or even in a specific house? Have you ever desired to be in a certain job or in a certain life situation, such as being married when you weren't? Have you ever hoped that God would call you to a specific ministry position, such as being a Bible teacher, overseas missionary or counselor?

When we give Christ control over our lives, He promises to lead us and arrange the events of our lives for the greatest possible good. Sometimes it might seem as if God is taking a long time to arrange those events, but He always has a reason for His timing. As He declared to the prophet Isaiah, "For my thoughts are not your thoughts, neither are your ways my ways" (Isaiah 55:8). Today, we will look at surrendering our destinations to God. He knows where He wants to take us. The encouragement for us is to let go, rest in Him and let Him guide our futures.

Have you ever hoped that the Lord would guide you to a specific location or position? If so, what was it that you wanted?

_____

_____

_____

It's been said that no new beginning can first happen without an end. Read Genesis 12:1-8. What three things was Abram called to leave behind (see v. 1)?

_____

_____

_____

What was God's promise to Abram if He followed Him and made this new beginning (see v. 2)?

_____

_____

_____

Have you, like Abram, ever had to leave something behind in order to make a new beginning? If so, what was it?

_____

_____

_____

Note that God didn't specifically describe Abram's final destination. Have you ever started on a journey and not known the outcome? What did it feel like to take that step of faith and follow the Lord? What steps of faith do you need to take on this wellness journey?

_____

_____

_____

How did the Lord reveal Himself to Abram along the way during his journey (see vv. 6-8)?

_____

_____

_____

How might you have experienced the presence of God along the way during your journey?

_____

_____

_____

The writer of Hebrews describes Abram's journey of faith in Hebrews 11:8-15. This passage suggests that people often do not see the destinations they had hoped (see v. 13). Why do you think God allows this?

_____

_____

_____

_____

> *Oh Lord, my life is in Your hands. You have a purpose*
> *for everything. I rest in Your guidance and provision. Amen.*

Day 3 — RELEASING OUR SECURITY

God, You have given me wisdom to know how to live a balanced life, but still my ultimate security comes from You. I trust in You. Amen.

We all want security. In fact, psychologists tell us that with the exception of significance, it is the most important life foundation for which we search. Security is the degree of protection we feel against danger and loss. Simply put, security means that we don't feel shaken. With security, our lives are stable. They are not necessarily predictable, but they are not rocked by events. Our lives feel safe.

God always invites us to lead lives of wisdom. It's not wrong to purchase insurance, put up a fence around our backyards or fasten our seat belts when we drive to town. Yet there is nothing we can do to make our lives completely secure. The only real security we have is in knowing that our lives are in God's hands. This is what we will look at today.

Begin today's study by reading the story of Gideon in Judges 6:11-16. At the time this story takes place, the Israelites had again faltered in their devotion to the Lord. A semi-nomadic group known as the Midianites had begun to harass them and invade their land, ruining their crops and killing their livestock. When the Israelites called out to God for deliverance, He began to put His plans in place for Gideon.

Why was Gideon threshing wheat in a winepress when the angel of the Lord met him (see v. 1)?

_____

_____

_____

What did the angel say to Gideon? What was Gideon's response (see vv. 12-13)?

_____

_____

_____

Notice that when Gideon questioned God about the hardships his nation was going through, God did not answer his question directly. Instead, He gave Gideon his marching orders. What were they (see v. 14)?

_____

_____

_____

Much like Moses, Gideon complained that he was not up to the task. He felt insignificant because of his birth and position. However, the Lord indicated that he was secure. What was Gideon's security (see v. 16)?

_____

_____

_____

What reasons might you give for not feeling secure? What knowledge do you have that everything is truly secure? (Hint: see Psalm 16:8.)

_____

_____

_____

_____

On three separate occasions, Gideon asks for God to affirm that He is truly with him. First, he asks God for a sign when he brings an offering (see v. 16). Later, he leaves a wool fleece on the threshing floor and asks God to make it covered with dew, but leave the ground dry. When God does this, Gideon then asks Him to make the fleece dry, but leave the ground covered with dew (see vv. 36-40). How have you tested the Lord in a similar manner? What was the result?

_____

_____

_____

_____

Read Judges 7:1-8. In this passage, the Lord tells Gideon to fight a battle. Gideon begins the battle with a strong army of many thousands of men, but through a series of events, God reduces the army to only 300 men. What reason did the Lord have for reducing the size of Gideon's army?

_____

_____

_____

What was Gideon's and Israel's ultimate security?

_____

_____

_____

As you conclude today's study, realize that like Gideon, God has promised to be with you as you fight the battle to maintain physical, emotional and spiritual health. Have you seen evidence of this security in your life? If you haven't, ask God to reveal His power in your life. If you have, say a prayer of thanksgiving to God for His provision and His care.

Lord, You are my rock and my provider. You are my security. My life is in Your hands. Today, I want to rest in Your guidance and provision. Amen.

RELEASING OUR FINANCES

Lord God, help me understand what I need to know about my finances so that they do not control me. I release them into Your care. Amen.

For many of us, finances are a regular concern. We dream about having more money. We wonder if we'll have enough money when we retire. We worry day to day if we're going to be able to pay our bills at the end of each month. Money is just a part of life.

The Bible actually has a lot to say about money. In fact, Jesus talked more about money than He did anything else, with the exception of the kingdom of God. Of His 39 parables, 11 talk about money. And 1 out of every 7 verses in the Gospel of Luke deal with money.

Paul also talks about money. In 1 Timothy 6:10, he writes this strong warning: "For the love of money is the root of all kinds of evil. Some people, eager for money, have wandered from the faith and pierced themselves with many griefs." Note here that Paul isn't saying that money itself is wrong. But the love of it is.

Let's take a look at some of these ideas more closely. In the following table, look up the proverb listed in the left-hand column, then summarize what it says about money in the right-hand column.

Proverb	What this proverb says about money
Proverbs 1:19	
Proverbs 10:16	
Proverbs 11:28	
Proverbs 22:7	

Read Luke 12:22-26. In this passage, what is Jesus saying about money?

_____

_____

_____

Does Jesus mean that we should never think about money, because God handles it all? Or is He saying something more about our attitude toward money here? Explain.

_____

_____

_____

In Psalm 50:10, the Lord says, "Every animal of the forest is mine, and the cattle on a thousand hills." How would this verse apply to giving Christ control over your money?

_____

_____

_____

In Philippians 4:19, Paul writes, "God will meet all your needs according to his glorious riches in Christ Jesus." How might this verse apply to giving Christ control over your money?

_____

_____

_____

How does First Place 4 Health's foundational teaching in Matthew 6:33 reveal how you are to think and act concerning money?

_____

_____

_____

What might it look like to release control of your finances to the Lord?

_____

_____

_____

_____

To lead a healthy life, it is vital that we keep our lives in balance with Christ securely at the center. So as you conclude today's study, consider whether you have allowed money to throw any of your priorities out of balance. Spend some time in prayer and truly give control of your finances—and your worries—over to the Lord.

> *Lord, teach me what I need to know about money. Let me be wise about it and use if for good purposes, but let me never be enslaved to it. I release control over my finances to You. Amen.*

RELEASING OUR PASTS

Day 5

> *Lord God, You say in Your Word that all things are made new in Christ Jesus (see 2 Corinthians 5:17). Help me always to go forward with that perspective. Thank You for the work of the cross. Amen.*

Sometimes we would like to move forward into a new area of responsibility, balance or blessing, but the thought of where we've been, what we've done or what we've been through holds us back. In such situations, we feel weighed down by our past actions. It is hard to know how we can go forward when there is such a cloud of discouragement, guilt, heaviness or just plain *yuck* hanging over our heads.

Christ offers us a new way of looking at things. Because of the work He did on the cross, our past doesn't have to hold us back. He invites us to place our former lives firmly at the foot of the cross and let His blood wash over all of our yesterdays. That's exciting news. Today is a new day in Christ. Let's look at this idea in Scripture more closely.

Read John 1:12. If you've received Christ, you are a child of God. How should the truth of this new identity affect your life?

_____

_____

_____

Is there anything in your life that you would like to "start over"?

_____

_____

_____

_____

One verse that puts this thought into perspective is 2 Corinthians 5:17. Spend some time meditating on and praying through this verse, and then fill in the blanks as they apply to your life.

The Bible says that if anyone is in Christ, he or she is a new creation. That's me. So with confidence I can write _____ [your name goes here] is a new creation.

Scripture says that "the old has gone," and that means that I no longer need to be concerned about this in my past. Scripture says that "the new has come," and that means that I can now look forward to:

_____

_____

_____

If I am ever reminded about my past, or if my past keeps me from going forward, I will remind myself about this verse. Here's one phrase or sentence from 2 Corinthians 5:17 to help me remember this verse:

_____

_____

_____

Remember that the action of releasing your past to the Lord may be more complex than what we've covered today. Today is just intended to be a foundational lesson on releasing your past, and you may need the help of a counselor or a group of trusted friends to fully complete the process. You may also need to remind yourself of these truths more than once. So be patient in this process, and remember that the Lord is good.

Lord, the old has gone and the new has come. Thank You for making me a new creation. I release my past to You. Help me go forward with You. Amen.

REFLECTION AND APPLICATION

Day 6

Thank You, God, for helping me release my life to You. Amen.

This week, we've looked at allowing God to take the wheel of our lives: our calling, our destination, our security, our finances and our past. We've asked the questions, *What would it look like if we sought only His will for our lives? What would it look like if we stopped chasing our own ambitions? What would it look like if we truly "ceased striving" and lived as if we knew He was God (see Psalm 46:10)?*

Today, simply allow yourself to rest in His care. You may want to journal some thoughts about areas of your life that Christ is inviting you to yield to Him. Using the following prompts, write those thoughts in the space provided, or write them down in your prayer journal.

Lord Jesus, I sense You are inviting me to yield this area of my life to You . . .

_____

_____

_____

But I still feel this way about it . . .

_____

_____

_____

Help me to remember You say in Your Word that . . .

_____

_____

_____

Help me want to release this area to You. With Your help, I will do so and boldly say . . .

_____

_____

_____

Lord, I do want to release everything in my life to You. Please watch over me and let me experience Your presence in my life.

Day 7 — REFLECTION AND APPLICATION

Lord, thank You for the blessings in my life. All that I am and everything I have comes from You. I love You, Lord, and I want to follow You. Amen.

Take a moment and recall all of the characters in Scripture that we've studied this week. On Day One, we saw how Joseph surrendered his future to God. When he was sold into slavery and later languished in prison, it must have seemed as if God had forgotten him. But, in fact, God had everything under control. He was molding and shaping Joseph into the man He wanted him to become. On Day Two, we saw how Abram surrendered his destination to God. Abram had faith in the Lord and followed His direction, and the Lord fulfilled His promise and made Abram into a great and mighty nation.

On Day Three, we saw how Gideon surrendered his security to God. Not that he was overly bold about it—he doubted God's call and asked the Lord to perform a series of tests to confirm it. Yet in the end, he also had faith and followed the Lord. On Day Four, we examined how Jesus told us to surrender our finances to Him and not to "worry about your life, what you will eat; or about your body, what you will wear . . . [for] who of you by worrying can add a single hour to his life?" (Luke 12:22,25).

On Day Five, we explored how He calls us to give our pasts to Him and embrace the new creation that He has made us.

As you conclude this week's study, look at each of these areas in your own life. How have you released the control of your calling, your destination, your security, your finances and your past to the Lord? Write down one way that you have (or will) release control in each area.

My calling:

_____

_____

_____

My destination:

_____

_____

_____

My security:

_____

_____

_____

My finances:

_____

_____

_____

My past:

_____

_____

_____

Note
1. Susan Scott Krabacher, *Angels of a Lower Flight* (New York: Touchstone Books, 2007), p. 7.

Group Prayer Requests

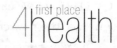

Today's Date: _____

Name	Request

Results

_____

_____

_____

_____

_____

_____

surrendering our words

SCRIPTURE MEMORY VERSE

*If anyone considers himself religious and yet
does not keep a tight rein on his tongue,
he deceives himself and his religion is worthless.*

JAMES 1:26

What we say reflects so much of what is inside of us. Words are like tools. In the hands of a trained craftsman, they can create things of beauty and inspiration. But in careless hands, they can bring despair and darkness.

James has quite a bit to say about the tongue in his epistle. In James 3:3-4, he compares the tongue to a bit in a horse's mouth or to the rudder of a ship. The bit and the rudder are small instruments, but they steer the horse or the ship wherever the rider or pilot wants them to go. In the same way, the tongue, though small, is a powerful part of the body. It has the power to direct us in life and to build up or to destroy.

For this reason, James wrote that the impact of our spiritual life can be neutralized if we fail to give Christ control over our words. It's not that we no longer have any responsibility in the matter, but rather that we now fully invite Christ's presence to impact what we say. Christ lives inside of us (see 2 Corinthians 13:5), and whenever we yield control of our lives to the Holy Spirit, God works in us "to will and to act according to his good purpose" (Philippians 2:13).

This week, we'll look more closely at what the Bible says about our speech. We'll examine some words that hurt and heal. We'll also gain insights into the potential for using words for God's glory.

WORDS, WORDS, WORDS

God, it is often so easy to speak before I consider the weight my words may have on another person. Help me to yield control of what I say to You. Amen.

Compared to giving Christ control over our actions, thoughts or emotions, it may seem less vital to give Him control over what we say. Yet, as we see in the epistle of James, the Bible speaks with great force and clarity about the importance of controlling our speech. Until we can control what comes out of our mouths, we will continue to be vulnerable to living a life out of balance. A chaotic mouth equals a chaotic life.

There is an interesting story told in the Bible about a man who had a problem keeping control over his tongue. Turn in your Bible to 1 Samuel 25:2-13. What two things does the Bible tell us about Nabal (see vv. 2-3)?

_____

_____

_____

At the time of this story, David was in hiding from King Saul and living out in the desert. He and his men had refrained from helping themselves to the animals in Nabal's flock, which they could have easily done. In return, now that it was shearing time—typically a time of feasting with much food to spare—David sent an envoy to Nabal to petition for some food. How does David phrase his request (see vv. 5-8)?

_____

_____

_____

How did the wealthy Nabal respond to the request (see vv. 10-11)?

_____

_____

_____

How did David respond when he heard Nabal's reply (see v. 13)?

_____

_____

_____

The story has a happy ending (at least for David). When Nabal's wife, Abigail, hears about the situation, she intercedes on her husband's behalf and convinces him not to attack. Later, when Nabal is feasting, his heart fails him and he becomes "like a stone" (v. 37). Ten days after that, Nabal dies, and David asks Abigail to become his wife. In the end, what does this story tell us about the power of our words?

_____

_____

_____

One of the first things that God wants us to transform as He works in our lives is our speech. After all, if God is really at work in our hearts, it should follow that our speech should demonstrate His righteous influence. Look up James 1:26, the memory verse for this week. What does this verse imply about people who call themselves Christians but who cannot control their tongues?

_____

_____

_____

Read Philippians 1:27. How might this verse apply to a changed life?

_____

_____

_____

Heavenly Father, You say that a word aptly spoken is like apples of gold in settings of silver (see Proverbs 25:11). Help me to be careful about my speech and use my words to build others up today. Amen.

THE POTENTIAL OF WORDS

Lord, help me to learn the discipline of keeping silent in order to listen to others. Help me to learn to use words that will bring comfort. Amen.

In 1666, the city of London was a disaster waiting to happen. The streets of the medieval city were narrow, and the buildings were constructed closely together. Adding to the problem, most of the structures were made from timber, plaster and pitch and filled with combustible materials such as tallow, straw and firewood.

In the early hours of September 2, 1666, a baker named Thomas Farriner failed to properly douse the ovens in his bakehouse. As a result, an ember blew out of one of the ovens and ignited some nearby straw. As the bakehouse went up in flames, embers spread to neighboring buildings, also setting them on fire. The fire soon spread to the warehouses packed with combustible materials on the Thames River, where it gained such strength that it could not be put out for four and a half days.

By the end of the ordeal, the fire had virtually leveled London. More than 13,000 houses had been destroyed, leaving up to 200,000 people homeless and destitute. The fire took out churches and many famous and important buildings. And it all started with a small spark.

Like an ember, a careless word can ignite a raging fire and ravage the lives of others. We have the potential to build up others with praise or hurt them with anger, bitterness or thoughtlessness. This is why we are instructed in Scripture to guard our tongues (see Psalm 141:3). Because words express our thoughts and ideas, our speech serves as a barometer of the spiritual pressure level of our hearts. Spoken words tend to reinforce our thoughts, so if we yield control over our thought life to the Lord, what comes out of our mouths will be more honoring to Him.

To begin today's study, take the following inventory of how well you control your tongue. As you read each statement, rate yourself on a scale of 0 to 10, with 0 being "never or hardly at all" and 10 being "most of the time, regularly or consistently."

_____ I remain silent when I know I should. God helps me know when I should and should not speak.

_____ I know when to stop talking.

_____ I'm a good listener.

_____ When another person is talking, I'm not thinking about what I'm going to say next.

_____ I tend to keep strong opinions to myself.

_____ I speak the truth to others, but I do so in love.

_____ I think I'm an encouraging person.

_____ One of my consistent goals is to build others up by what I say.

_____ I can set the tone in my house by what I say, so I consistently try to speak words that reflect comfort, encouragement, grace, humor and patience.

_____ **Total**

Scoring:
76-90: You have excellent control over your words.
51-75: You are mindful of what you say most of the time.
26-50: You could use some work in this area.
0-25: London is burning!

Read James 3:3-10. We looked at James' analogy of the bit and rudder in the introduction to this week's session, but what other analogy does James use here to describe the power and impact of the tongue (see v. 6)?

_____

_____

_____

How can the analogy of the bit, rudder and fire relate to the potentially positive impact of our words?

_____

_____

_____

James states all kinds of beasts, birds and serpents can be tamed (v. 7). What does he say can't be tamed? Why do you think he feels this way?

_____

_____

_____

What does he say about the dual nature of the tongue (see v. 9)? Why is this a problem for Christians?

_____

_____

_____

According to 1 Corinthians 2:13, what does Paul say is the source of our power when talking to others about Christ?

_____

_____

_____

Read Matthew 12:34-37. What implications do Jesus' words have for Christians?

_____

_____

_____

As you conclude today's session, can you describe a time when you believed the Holy Spirit gave you special words while speaking to someone about spiritual matters? How did that make you feel?

_____

_____

_____

Lord, I invite You, in the same manner as David did, to "set a guard over my mouth . . . [and] keep watch over the door of my lips" (Psalm 141:3). Amen.

WORDS TO AVOID

Heavenly Father, help me to always speak the truth in love, even when I am in situations where it may be difficult to do so. Amen.

The French philosopher Blaise Pascal once said, "Cold words freeze people, and hot words scorch them, and bitter words make them bitter, and wrathful words make them wrathful. Kind words also produce their image on men's souls; and a beautiful image it is. They soothe, and quiet, and comfort the hearer."

The Bible consistently encourages us to use kind words with one another. It also warns against many types of words, heart actions and behaviors that are inappropriate, harmful or that lead to imbalance. Some of these include quarreling, lying and flattery. These three ways of interacting with people are all ways that we can use words to stir up trouble—both for ourselves and for the people around us.

Our invitation is always to be people who produce kind words that soothe, quiet and comfort the hearer. Today, we will look more closely at some of these ideas as found in Scripture.

Proverbs 12:18 states, "Reckless words pierce like a sword, but the tongue of the wise brings healing." How have you experienced the truth of this verse in your own life or in the lives of others?

_____

_____

_____

_____

Two types of negative speech—gossip and slander—can make deep cuts and wound our friendships. What does Paul tell us to do about slander in Ephesians 4:31?

_____

_____

_____

What does he say about the seriousness of gossip and slander in Romans 1:29-30?

_____

_____

_____

Quarreling and flattery are two other types of negative speech we are urged to avoid. Whenever we quarrel, we lose our focus on the truth and let our emotions drive our decisions. When we flatter, we use truths and half-truths to manipulate others. Our words plant seeds of discord and destruction in our relationships, and that ultimately leads to trouble. What do the following passages say about quarrelling or flattery.

Romans 16:17-18

_____

_____

_____

Colossians 3:8-9

_____

_____

James 4:1-2

_____

_____

_____

So, how do we prevent this misuse of the tongue and avoid using this type of negative speech? In Psalm 120:1, the psalmist offers one solution: "I call on the LORD in my distress, and he answers me." As you close today's session, think about this solution and how you can apply it to your life this week in a practical way.

Lord, help me to avoid engaging in gossip, slander, flattery or any other type
of language that brings strife. Be at the center of my conversations. Amen.

WORDS THAT WORSHIP IN ALL SITUATIONS

Day 4

Lord God, help my lips to continually bring You glory—and not just
during times of corporate worship, but every day and at every moment.
Let my words continually reflect Your righteous character. Amen.

One of our primary goals should always be to know when to keep silent and when to speak. In addition, Christ invites us to rid our speech of words that stir up trouble or hurt people and build good relationships with our words. Yet our words do even more, for it is through our speech that we worship God in prayer. Throughout the psalms, David and other writers use words to exalt, praise, thank and worship God.

The following are examples of the psalmists using words to worship, praise, exalt and thank the Lord. After reading the verses, choose the word that best describes the theme of each one.

_____	Psalm 18:49	a.	Worship
_____	Psalm 30:12	b.	Praise
_____	Psalm 34:3	c.	Exaltation
_____	Psalm 100:2	d.	Thanks

What instruction does Paul give to believers in Ephesians 5:19-20 concerning praise and worship?

_____

_____

_____

Paul tells us that we are to give thanks to God the Father in all things, and he often backed up his words with the example of his life. Read

Acts 16:16-26. What was the initial situation that distressed Paul, and what did he do as a result (see vv. 16-18)?

_____

_____

_____

How did the owners of the girl react to Paul's actions (see vv. 19-21)?

_____

_____

_____

Paul and Silas were flogged and thrown into prison. Certainly, this was not a pleasant situation for either of them to be in. But what do we see them doing in verse 25?

_____

_____

_____

_____

Paul truly praised God in all situations—and so can each of us. In closing, read Psalm 136. Note the repeated line throughout: _His love endures forever._ In the space below, write your own prayer, psalm or song to the Lord using phrases of worship, praise and thanksgiving from your own life. Intersperse your phrases with the line _"His love endures forever."_

_____

_____

_____

_____

_____

Heavenly Father, may my words always be in praise and honor of Your holy name. May I praise You in all situations, even when I am facing the dark storm clouds of life. I give thanks to You for the many blessings You give. Amen.

WORDS THAT CREATE RELATIONSHIPS

Lord, let me boldly speak the words that others need to hear. Give direction to my thoughts and tongue so that I would speak the wisdom of God. Amen.

Our words can build relationships with God and can also become tools for building relationships with people. Proverbs 15:4 illustrates this truth in both a positive and a negative light when is states, "The tongue that brings healing is a tree of life, but a deceitful tongue crushes the spirit."

Have you ever considered what you say as a vehicle for bringing healing to others? Just as Jesus' words brought healing to the bodies and souls of His early followers, we are invited to bring healing to the lives of the people around us with the words we speak. We have tremendous power to *heal* and *help* with what we say. Let's look at this idea more closely today.

The verses in the left-hand column in the following table all refer to words that build relationships. Read each passage, and then in the right-hand column write how following the instructions in the passage would enable you to help and heal others.

Verse	How this would help and heal another person
Ephesians 1:15-16	
Colossians 3:13	
Colossians 3:16	
1 Thessalonians 5:11	
1 Thessalonians 5:14	
1 Peter 2:17	

Now think of some recent conversations you have had with people you know. This could be an acquaintance, a family member or even another person in your First Place 4 Health group. Circle any words in the right-hand column in the table above that could be used to describe what was said. Did you find that you used a lot of these words to heal, strengthen, build up, minister and help these individuals? If not, what could you have done differently?

_____

_____

_____

_____

You should be encouraged if you find that the majority of what you have said helps others. However, if you discover that you have used negative words to interact with people recently, don't despair. Just confess to God that you have not been the best at using your words in this area. Ask Him to guide you in your dealings with others so that you can use more encouraging and healing words.

To conclude today's session, read or recite Philippians 4:8, the memory verse from our Week Four study. Then write down some ways below in which you can apply this verse to your life and to what you say.

_____

_____

_____

_____

Heavenly Father, let me be a minister of Your peace and glory today by the words I say. I give you control over my speech. Please fill me to the full measure with all the goodness of Your Holy Spirit. Let my words always bring honor to You. Thank You, Lord. Amen.

REFLECTION AND APPLICATION

*Heavenly Father, as Your Word says, let my words be like a honeycomb,
sweet to the soul and healing to the bones (see Proverbs 16:24). Please bless
my words today and use them to help others. Thank You, Lord. Amen.*

As the proverb states, "The tongue has the power of life and death, and those who love it will eat its fruit" (Proverbs 18:21). In this week's study, we looked at the power of our words and how they can be used to tear down as well as build up. They can heal or cause great pain. They can comfort or bring great sorrow. Words are our primary means of communication with others, and whether those words are written, spoken, or implied, they will always convey our thoughts, ideas, plans, hopes and attitudes.

As we discussed in our Day Two study, it only takes a spark to ignite a raging fire. Maybe you've caused damage in your relationships with a word spoken in carelessness, frustration or anger. Perhaps you've set them ablaze like the great fire in London and you don't see any way to restore life to that friendship that once flourished.

Yet there is something to remember about the great fire in London: after it was over, builders were commissioned to redesign the city. Within the span of just a few years, more than 9,000 houses and public buildings had been completed, including the famous St. Paul's Cathedral, today one of the great national landmarks of the city.

God gives us the opportunity to experience His power whenever we speak. He can restore our relationships if we invite Him to take control of our words and actions. When we use what we have learned in the Bible and simply tell others about these things, God promises to bless what we say and how those words are used in the lives of others.

So spend some time today journaling about your speech patterns and how you use words. Allow God to take control of what you say and how you say it. Is there any area in which you would like to improve? Is there any situation that you have recently experienced that you want to thank Him for giving you the wisdom to handle correctly?

Write your thoughts in the space below or in your prayer journal.

_____

_____

_____

_____

_____

Lord, let the words of my mouth and the meditation of my heart be pleasing in Your sight, O Lord, my Rock and my Redeemer (see Psalm 19:14). Amen.

Day
7

REFLECTION AND APPLICATION

Lord, let my words today communicate Your glory. Let me be filled with praise so that I may bless You and bless others. Amen.

A second focus this week has been to worship God with our speech. The Bible indicates that we can use the Word of God to teach, instruct, forgive, challenge, inspire, edify, affirm, honor, pardon and encourage others—and that any time we do these things, we reflect the character of a righteous God. That's worship, in a sense. It's showing God we respect Him and acknowledging the truth that's His. So today, let's use a few passages of Scripture to write out some prayers to the Lord. As you do so, spend some time focusing on His greatness and goodness.

Praise: Using the words of Psalm 9:1-2, write a prayer to God expressing gratitude for who He is.

_____

_____

_____

_____

Worship: Using the words of Psalm 95:6-7, write a prayer expressing your love to God.

_____

_____

_____

_____

_____

_____

Thanksgiving: Using the words of Psalm 118:29, write a prayer expressing gratitude for what God has done in your life.

_____

_____

_____

_____

_____

_____

Lord, I see the power of my words and I want to use them wisely for Your purposes. Today, simply, I give You control of my speech.

Group Prayer Requests

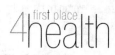

Today's Date: _____

Name	Request

Results

_____

_____

_____

_____

_____

how to let go of control

SCRIPTURE MEMORY VERSE
If anyone would come after me, he must deny himself and take up his cross daily and follow me.
LUKE 9:23

When it comes to giving Christ control of our lives, the big question that often stymies people is *how*. We recognize God's goodness and want to be people whose lives are yielded to Him, but we're unsure of how to proceed. What do we do? What steps do we take? How do we consistently rest in Him (see Hebrews 4:9-11), lean not on our own understanding (see Proverbs 3:5-6), cast our anxiety upon Him (see 1 Peter 5:7), and let Him take the lead (see Psalm 32:8)?

Fortunately, we have a God who never aims to make anything overly complicated. Jesus says, "Take my yoke upon you and learn from me, for I am gentle and humble in heart, and you will find rest for your souls" (Matthew 11:29). This is Christ's invitation for us to yield to Him. It doesn't need to be difficult.

NOT COMPLICATED, BUT NOT EASY

Day 1

Lord Jesus, Your commandments are always straightforward but sometimes difficult for me to follow. Help me to look to You for strength. Amen.

"If something is worth doing, it probably won't be easy." How many times have you heard people say something like this to you? Well, it's true. If you want to get a college degree, have a successful marriage, be a good parent or even be a good friend, the road ahead might be straightforward, but it won't always be easy.

As much as Jesus' call to us to take His yoke upon ourselves is straightforward, the path of discipleship isn't always easy to follow. Many of Christ's instructions contain elements of difficulty. For instance, "Love your neighbor as yourself" (Matthew 19:19). Have you ever been called to love someone who wasn't easy to love? Someone who was just argumentative and difficult to get along with? Jesus' instruction is straightforward, but it can be very challenging to follow.

Turn in your Bible to Luke 9:23, our memory verse for this week. In this verse, Jesus lays out three basic commitments that are part of following Him. What are those three commitments?

1. _____

_____

2. _____

_____

3. _____

_____

What are some of the most challenging aspects of being a Christian as you consider these three commitments?

_____

_____

_____

How might a person deny himself or herself? How might that person put aside his or her own wishes for the sake of a greater good?

_____

_____

_____

How might a person take up his or her cross? How might that person take up the call to love the world (see John 3:16) even though it brings pain and separation from loved ones—or even death?

_____

_____

_____

How might a person follow Christ? How might he or she seek to under-take the ministry of Jesus Christ in everyday life?

_____

_____

_____

Read Mark 12:29-31. According to this verse, what two components are foundational to all ministries?

_____

_____

_____

How do you define the word "ministry"?

_____

_____

_____

What sort of things do you enjoy doing to demonstrate Christ's love to others? How could you view this as your "ministry"?

_____

_____

_____

Father God, what is Your call on my life? It is to love and serve You,
and to love and serve others. Help me to do this. Amen.

Day 2   STAYING CLOSE

Lord Jesus, thank You that You desire to spend time with me in fellowship.
Help me to always abide in You and live in Your Word. Amen.

When you wake up each morning, what are some of your first thoughts? If you're like most people, you're thinking about what you need to do for the day, or about how well you just slept (or didn't sleep), or how quickly you can get to that first cup of coffee.

What if your first thought each morning was of the Person you're invited to love most of all: the Lord? What would happen if the first thing you did was reconnect with the God of the universe? People who create the healthy habit of connecting with the Lord each day find that life tends to fall into order that way. They recognize that each day is something the Lord made. Not only are His mercies new every morning, but He also invites us to rejoice in each day as a gift of His creation.

The scriptural word for closeness to God is "abide." Christ invites us to abide with Him. This simply means that we stay close to Him. Each day, we connect with Him through His Word and prayer. This is one way that we give control of our lives to Christ—by abiding in Him. Today we will examine this idea in more detail.

In John 15:5, Jesus said, "I am the vine; you are the branches. If a man remains in me and I in him, he will bear much fruit; apart from me you can do nothing." What was Jesus saying in using this analogy about what our relationship should be with Him?

_____

_____

_____

What did He mean by the phrase "apart from me you can do nothing"?

_____

_____

_____

Read John 8:31-32. What action is necessary for staying close to Christ?

_____

_____

_____

Jesus said that His truth sets people free. How have you experienced that freedom in your own life? Give a few examples.

_____

_____

_____

Think about your current devotional life. What habits and heart attitudes do you have that enable you to stay close to the Lord?

_____

_____

_____

Is this what you would like your devotional life to be like? If not, what will you do to change the situation?

_____

_____

_____

_____

Some people view spending time with Christ each day in His Word as a challenge. To them, it sort of feels like going to the dentist—it's good for you, but not much fun. Others see it not as a "discipline" at all but more as a relationship. To them, it's more like having coffee with a good friend. As you conclude today's study, think about how you view your relationship with Christ. What analogy might help you in this area?

Father God, apart from You, I can do nothing. Let me
always stay close to You and abide in Your love. Amen.

PRAYING ALWAYS

Jesus, I want to be in contact with You as I go throughout my day. Fill me each day with Your presence and help me to always be mindful of You. Amen.

Martin Luther King, Jr. once said, "To be a Christian without prayer is no more possible than to be alive without breathing." Prayer is just a natural part of the Christian's life. It is simply talking to God, and it can happen anytime, anywhere and with any words—or with no words at all.

Some people view prayer as a formal event. They think it needs to be done in a specific place (usually a church) and performed by a professional clergy. Others view prayer as a discipline. It's a duty, something that needs to be done and checked off a spiritual checklist. Sure, it's good for people, but there's not much joy in it. Christ offers a different perspective. He invites us to continually pray to Him in close relationship. Let's take a look at this idea more closely.

Read Ephesians 1:7 and 2:13-14. What work has Christ done for us?

_____

_____

_____

_____

Turn in your Bible to Hebrews 4:14-16. With what attitude does Christ invite us to approach Him in prayer?

_____

_____

_____

Read 1 John 5:14-15. According to this passage, what confidence is ours?

_____

_____

_____

_____

What is the promise Jesus gave us regarding prayer in John 15:7?

_____

_____

_____

_____

What are the two conditions Jesus gives for this promise?

_____

_____

_____

_____

What is the promise and the condition for answered prayer found in Matthew 21:22 and Mark 11:24?

_____

_____

_____

_____

Read 1 Thessalonians 5:16-18. How does Paul encourage us to pray in this passage?

_____

_____

_____

_____

As you conclude today's study, reflect on how you typically view prayer. Is it more a duty or discipline, or more a relationship with Someone you love?

> *Heavenly Father, thank You that I can always talk to You. I approach You boldly and with reverence. Help me to know Your perfect will as I read the Bible and to pray with confidence in accordance with Your will. Amen.*

SPENDING TIME WITH OTHERS

Lord Jesus, help me to develop the friendships I need to bring me closer to
You. Please bring godly people into my circle of friends who will speak
Your words of wisdom into my life. Amen.

Another way to give control of your life to Christ is by spending time with people who will bring you closer to Him. The word in Scripture often used to describe this is "fellowship," which simply means friendships with a spiritual purpose. When we fellowship with other believers, we share our common experiences and build one another up in Christ.

If you have been in First Place 4 Health for any length of time, you undoubtedly comprehend the value of fellowship. It is comforting to have people around you who understand the struggles you are facing and are there for you when you feel weak in a particular area. They have often been where you are now, and they can impart the godly wisdom you need in your life to help you persevere. Likewise, there are people in your group who need your help and support, and God can work through you to be a powerful force in that person's life. Fellowship is a two-way street.

One of the most fascinating depictions of fellowship in the Bible is that of the Early Church. In Acts 2:42-47, to what did the believers devote themselves (see v. 42)?

_____

_____

_____

_____

What was unique about the way these believers took care of each other (see vv. 44-45)?

_____

_____

_____

_____

What did they do each day that strengthened their fellowship?

_____

_____

_____

What occurred as a result of how they led their lives (see v. 47)?

_____

_____

_____

Those in the Early Church lived lives that reflected Christ's love, and that was attractive to many people in the culture of the time—just as it is today. Read 1 Thessalonians 5:11. What is one way to love others?

_____

_____

_____

Read 2 Corinthians 1:3-4. According to this passage, what benefits are found in close Christian friendships?

_____

_____

_____

Read John 15:13. What are some practical ways we can live out this verse in everyday life?

_____

_____

_____

What activities are (or are not) involved in true Christian fellowship?

_____

_____

_____

In John 13:34-35, Jesus commanded us to love one another. How can we do as Jesus commanded and invite others into our fellowship—even those who are difficult to love?

_____

_____

_____

God, I commit my friendships to You. Teach me how to give love more abundantly and to receive love as I fellowship with others. Amen.

Day 5 — BRINGING PEOPLE ONE STEP CLOSER

Lord Jesus, let me be a minister and a servant to others. Live and act through me so I can continually bring others one step closer to Christ. Amen.

As Christians, we know that Jesus commanded us to share the gospel with others. Yet most of us, if we're are honest about it, tend to dread evangelism. Although it's something we're sure we need to do, well . . . uh . . . we don't know what to say, or . . . it's not our spiritual gift, or . . . uh . . . it just feels too awkward to go up to people and ask them which section they're going to spend eternity in—smoking or non-smoking.

There are a million reasons Christians give for not witnessing about Christ, and frankly, many of those reasons are legitimate. Now, that may sound like a cop-out to you, but it's true: evangelism, as we so often define it, is strange to us because we live in a culture in which people seldom have deep conversations with anyone unless they know that person very well. Think of it this way: You wouldn't walk up to a stranger and say, "Hey, friend, I know a great stylist that can help you with that horrible hairdo you've got." That other person would get offended—or run—even if what you were about to tell him or her would actually help.

So let's take the pressure out of it and define true evangelism as bringing people one step closer to Christ. It's not that we reduce the message of the cross, but the real work of evangelism is always done by the Holy Spirit. He draws all people to Himself (see John 6:44), and our task is to be available to His moving. Usually, our call is simply to act authentically and talk to people in natural ways about what it means to have a relationship with Christ. We're also called to minister in practical ways—to be the hands and feet of Christ to a world that needs to see Him.

Read 2 Corinthians 5:11-15. According to Paul, what is our primary motivation for evangelism (see v. 11)?

_____

_____

_____

What should compel us to tell others about Christ (see v. 14)?

_____

_____

_____

What does this look like in your life? How does your love for Christ prompt you to tell or show others about Christ?

_____

_____

_____

Read Matthew 28:18-20. What is Jesus telling His disciples to do?

_____

_____

_____

People often mistakenly read the command in this passage as "to go." But in fact, the correct phrasing is, "as you go, make disciples." The real command is to make disciples. How does one make disciples?

_____

_____

_____

In Matthew 4:19, Jesus says, "Come, follow me . . . and I will make you fishers of men." What did Jesus mean by the phrase "fishers of men"?

_____

_____

_____

In Matthew 25:40, Jesus says, "I tell you the truth, whatever you did for one of the least of these brothers of mine, you did for me." As you conclude today's session, think about what it means to be the "hands and feet" of Christ in the world today. Give some practical examples.

_____

_____

_____

God, let me be available to minister to others. Let me authentically speak to others about Your love and show them love by my actions. Amen.

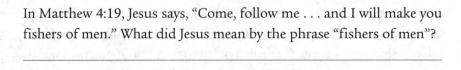

Day 6

REFLECTION AND APPLICATION

Heavenly Father, You ask that I give control of all that I am to You—heart, mind, body and spirit. Today I will give of my time and exercise the wonderful body that You created and called good. Amen.

In this week's study, we looked at practical ways that we can give control to Christ. We discussed how we can give of our time and commit to spending moments of each day in the Word, in prayer, in fellowship and in sharing the gospel with others. Today, we are going to put some of these things into practice and get some exercise in the process.

It's time to put on your shoes and do some walking. You have several choices for how you can do this exercise. First, you can engage in fellowship by calling up another person whom you may not know well and inviting them to go walking with you. As you walk, discuss some of the principles that you learned this week and what Christ is doing in your life. Or, you can make this a personal exercise and spend some time in prayer. As you walk, just talk to God about your day and thank Him for the glory of His creation that you see around you.

If you would like to spend additional time in the Word, use this time to memorize some of the verses we've discussed during this week's study. Matthew 21:22, Mark 11:24 and John 15:7 are excellent verses to memorize. When you hold verses like these in your heart, any stronghold that threatens to overtake your life is just waiting to be defeated by the Holy Spirit.

O Lord, help me as I seek to continually give You control over my life. I trust in You forever, for You, my Lord, are the Rock eternal. Amen.

REFLECTION AND APPLICATION   Day 7

Lord, I want to follow You even when the way is difficult at times. Help me to never lose sight of Your goodness. Amen.

This week's memory verse said: "If anyone would come after me, he must deny himself and take up his cross daily and follow me" (Luke 9:23). We looked at three commitments taken from this verse: (1) denying ourselves, (2) taking up our cross, and (3) following Christ. Today, spend some time in prayer, asking the Lord to give you insight into this week's verse and to help you to live this verse out daily. You may want to write out your prayer in your prayer journal or use the prompts below.

O Lord God, Your way is perfect and Your Word is flawless. You are my shield, and I take refuge in You (see Psalm 18:30).

Thank You God, that You know Your sheep. You have given me eternal life. No one can snatch me out of Your hand (see John 10:27-29).

Father, because I am in Christ, the devil has no hold on me (see John 14:30).

Conclude by writing in your prayer journal any thoughts you had from this week that will help you grow closer to the Lord.

Group Prayer Requests

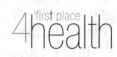

Today's Date: _____

Name	Request

Results

_____

_____

_____

_____

_____

_____

a community of encouragement

SCRIPTURE MEMORY VERSE

Let us consider how we may spur one another on toward love and good deeds. Let us not give up meeting together, as some are in the habit of doing, but let us encourage one another—and all the more as you see the Day approaching.

HEBREWS 10:24-25

Winston Churchill once said, "I am not a pillar of the church, but a buttress since I support it from without rather than from within." Sometimes, leading a Christian life in isolation is an enticing thought. And certainly there are times when we need to go off and spend some alone time to recharge. In fact, Jesus often did this: "Very early in the morning, while it was still dark, Jesus got up, left the house and went off to a solitary place, where he prayed" (Mark 1:35).

Yet far too many of us try to live a balanced life without the support of others. Truly, the Christian life is not meant to be experienced apart from community. God designed Christians to be interdependent and bound together through their relationships with Jesus Christ.

We looked at the value of having fellowship in Day Four of last week's study, but this week we will look at what it takes to have authentic friendships and the benefits we can receive when we connect our lives with others. We will explore how godly friendships can give us courage and help us see the blind spots in our lives. We will also see how when our friends speak the truth in love, it can move us out of a spiritual rut and get us back on track. In the end, we are all in this journey together.

AUTHENTIC FRIENDSHIPS

O Lord Jesus, let me be authentic with others and open to those in
my community of friends. I pray that You would use my friendships
to strengthen my walk with You. Amen.

As the world becomes more crowded and the pace of life accelerates,
we've become used to being surrounded by people. Yet at the same time,
we are seldom truly interacting with people or connecting authentically
with one another. We long to be accepted and loved by others. Personal
relationships are essential to healthy spiritual development. Without a
network of love and support, our lives can easily slip out of balance.

Read 1 Thessalonians 2:6-12. How does Paul describe his role as a spiritual father to his Christian friends (see v. 7)?

_____

_____

_____

_____

What does Paul say that indicates he had authentic friendships with
these believers (see v. 8)?

_____

_____

_____

_____

Have you ever participated in a group where the people shared biblical
truths but did not share about their personal lives? If so, what was that
like? How did it make you feel?

_____

_____

_____

_____

Have you ever been part of a community in which a spiritual father or mother or the group responded to you as Paul did with his friends (see vv. 7,11)? Describe the situation.

_____

_____

_____

If you allowed the image of a father or mother to guide your interactions with other Christians, how would you interact differently than you do now?

_____

_____

_____

Turn to James 5:16. What does this verse instruct Christians to do?

_____

_____

_____

What does this imply about the nature of the friendships we should have in our community of believers?

_____

_____

_____

Sharing genuine concern for others is a way to combat discouragement and downfall in our lives. When we are open with others and confess our faults—and don't allow pride to get in the way—everyone in the fellowship is strengthened. Sharing our needs, shortcomings, love, encouragement, sympathy and testimony with others can give us the strong supporting foundation we need to give control of our lives to Christ and live a balanced life.

If you have difficulty sharing with a group, find a close friend with whom you feel comfortable and talk openly with him or her. In many cases, sensitive issues should be shared in a private setting with a person who is trained and equipped to help deal with such problems. Perhaps one way to apply the instruction in James 5:16 is to say to others who share their hurts and failures, "God has forgiven you, God loves you, and so do we."

Thank You, Lord, for the love and acceptance of Christian friends, through whom I can experience Your unconditional love. Help me to become a loving and supportive friend to others. Amen.

Day 2

A PLACE TO FIND COURAGE

Lord, please grant me the courage—and encouragement—I need today to give You control over my life. Thank You for your righteous character. Amen.

The pressure of everyday life can drain away our courage. Like Joshua in the Old Testament, we constantly need to hear the words, "Be strong and courageous. Do not be terrified; do not be discouraged, for the LORD your God will be with you wherever you go" (Joshua 1:9). Discouragement leaves us vulnerable to sin. When we feel there is no reason to keep trying, we are more likely to move in negative directions or succumb to temptations. We need regular infusions of encouragement to face life.

Meeting regularly with a trusted group of friends can provide us with the encouragement we need to overcome spiritual imbalance and yield control of our lives to Christ. Our Christian walk requires constant support and accountability from our trusted friends. The good news is that success is possible—with God's help and our community of believers.

The book of Acts tells us about a man named Joseph who was such an encourager that the apostles actually called him "Barnabas," or "Son of Encouragement" (see Acts 4:36). Throughout Acts, we see examples of his generosity and all of the work he did to strengthen the resolve of the believers in the Early Church.

Read Acts 11:19-24. What was the situation that had caused the believers to disperse from Jerusalem (see v. 19)?

_____

_____

_____

What was happening in Antioch that had come to the attention of the apostles in Jerusalem (see vv. 20-21)?

_____

_____

_____

How did Barnabas respond? What does this say about his character?

_____

_____

_____

How can you be a "Barnabas" to someone today?

_____

_____

_____

In 2 Timothy 4:2, Paul gives Timothy instruction for becoming a more effective minister to his flock. How can the last part of this verse apply to you in a small group situation?

_____

_____

_____

Encouragement is one of the greatest gifts that Christians can give each other. The following verses provide some insights into how we should give and receive encouragement. Read each verse, and then complete the missing phrase.

- Romans 1:11-12: Use your spiritual _____ to encourage each other.
- Romans 15:4: God uses the _____ to encourage you and give you hope.
- Romans 15:5: It is _____ who will encourage you.
- 1 Thessalonians 5:11: We are to encourage and _____ each other up.
- 1 Thessalonians 5:14: Encourage the _____ and help the weak.
- Titus 1:9: Encourage others with _____ doctrine.
- Hebrews 10:25: Encourage one another as you _____ together.

As you conclude today's study, think of some practical ways that you can encourage those in your life. Perhaps a person in your First Place 4 Health group is struggling to maintain a healthy lifestyle and would benefit from receiving an email or phone call encouraging him or her to stay on track. Maybe there is someone at work who is feeling discouraged and could benefit from some kind words. Or maybe someone you know is launching out on a new endeavor and could use your prayers and support. Whatever the situation, commit this week to reach out to that person and build him or her up.

Thank You, Lord, for giving me Christian friends who support me.
Please use me to help others in reaching their goals. Amen.

Day 3 — HELP WITH BLIND SPOTS

O Lord, let me honestly look at Your Word today and honestly look at my life. Let me see any spiritual "blind spots" that have crept into my life. Amen.

Doctors tell us that a "blind spot," also known as a *scotoma*, is an area in our field of vision where our eyes cannot detect any objects. More often, however, we think of a blind spot in connection with driving in our cars. A blind spot is any area of the road that we cannot see while looking through either the rear-view mirror or side mirrors. If we don't check those blind spots before we switch lanes on a road, we run the risk of slamming into a car that has pulled up beside us.

One of the main reasons we need the support of Christian friends is to detect spiritual blind spots. These are areas of life, spiritually and emotionally, where something has crept us beside us that we do not see clearly. For many reasons, our perspective of these things becomes distorted and what we perceive to be reality is not accurate. In the same way that driving with an inaccurate map creates problems, so too living with blind spots complicates life. Let's take a look at this more closely today.

Read Galatians 6:2-5. What instructions did Paul give the Galatians?

_____

_____

_____

_____

Have you ever had a situation where a friend helped you with a blind spot? Describe that situation.

_____

_____

_____

_____

How can the verses in Galatians be applied to the idea of friends helping us with our blind spots?

_____

_____

_____

_____

In Matthew 7:1-5, Jesus also addressed the problem of blind spots. What does Jesus say about judging others (see vv. 1-2)?

_____

_____

_____

Have you ever judged someone, only to discover later that what you thought you saw so clearly in his or her life was actually an issue in your own life? If so, what did you learn from that situation?

_____

_____

_____

_____

Why is it typically easier to see the "specks" in other people's eyes while overlooking the "planks" in our eyes (see vv. 3-5)?

_____

_____

_____

How does taking the time to remove the plank from your own eye prepare you to help with the speck in another person's eye?

_____

_____

_____

_____

Judging others before we look at ourselves may cause us to be overconfident in our lives. Jesus' invitation is for us to test our own actions first, confess our sins, and then go to our brothers and sisters and speak to them in love. Our motivation should always be to encourage that person and lead him or her to restoration. When a group of Christian friends love each other enough to gently deal with one another's blind spots, great spiritual growth can occur. One of the greatest gifts we can give each other is clearer spiritual vision.

God, I ask that You reveal my blind spots to me, no matter how painful the process may be, and give me the opportunity to help others gently remove things from their lives that are hindering their spiritual growth. Amen.

STUCK IN A LOOP

Lord Jesus, if I've been stuck in any way, help me get back on track.
You are good, and I thank You for Your guidance. Amen.

When God called Moses to lead the Israelites out of Egypt, He promised to lead them to the Promised Land. He performed miraculous works in the form of plagues to "encourage" Pharaoh to let His people go. He led them through the Red Sea and appeared to them as a cloud by day and a pillar of fire at night.

But the people still grumbled and complained. They faltered at times and worshipped some of the gods they had come to know in Egypt. And when they arrived at the Promised Land, they heard reports of giants in the land and rebelled against Moses. As a result, they had to wander aimlessly in the desert for 40 years.

As Christians, we may occasionally get stuck in such "spiritual loops." Although we have witnessed the power of God, we just can't seem to get past a particular issue. So we wander in meandering circles, going no place in particular. We have lost our way. When this happens, how do we break the cycle to get out of this loop?

This is where the encouragement and support of our brothers and sisters in the Lord comes into play. Because we all have a tendency to lose direction or motivation at times, God invites us to connect with other Christians who can help us get moving in the right direction once again. Let's take a look at this idea more closely today.

Read Hebrews 3:7-13. This passage provides an excellent summary of the spiritual problems the Israelites experienced and how it led to them getting stuck in a loop (literally). According to this passage, why was God angry with this generation of the Israelites (see vv. 8-10)?

_____

_____

_____

_____

What was the consequence for their actions (see v. 11)?

_____

_____

_____

What does the writer of Hebrews say we are to do to help others stay out of such spiritual loops (see vv. 12-13)?

_____

_____

_____

Read this week's memory verse again (Hebrews 10:24-25). In practical terms, what are we to help others do?

_____

_____

_____

There may have been times when your spiritual life seemed to be going nowhere or you just couldn't motivate yourself to do what you needed to do. Often, a friend or someone close to you will notice discouragement in your life and will say or do the thing you need the most to get you going again. Think about such a time in your life. Who helped you, and what did that person say or do to help you get back on the right track?

_____

_____

_____

Without ongoing support and encouragement, we may stagnate in our Christian walk. Rather than growing in love and living the principles of our faith, we become comfortable or continue in harmful or imbalanced patterns of living. We need Christian friends who care enough to speak the truth in love to us—friends who love us enough to say, "Isn't it about time you got moving again?"

We also need to be willing to follow God's direction when we notice that someone in our circle of trusted friends needs a word of support or motivation. We need to be willing to step out and challenge that person to really look at what is going on in his or her life and move forward. As God directs us, we can encourage that friend in such a way that it will move him or her in their spiritual development.

As you conclude today's study, think about what you can do to spur or encourage spiritual growth in your circle of friends.

> *Heavenly Father, please bring people into my life who will encourage me in my spiritual walk. Likewise, help me be the friend I need to be. Use me to help other Christians have a right heart attitude toward Christ. Amen.*

PRAYING WITH OTHERS

Day 5

> *Lord Jesus, thank You for the friendships I have. Thank You that we can meet together to worship and praise You and bring our requests to You. Let us dwell in Your presence, for it is there we find light and life. Amen.*

In his book *How to Pray When You Don't Know What to Say*, Elmer Towns provides the following insight about the benefits of praying with other believers: "Jesus made an incredible promise to us that if we agree with each other in prayer, the answer will come. 'I tell you that if two of you agree about anything you ask for, it will be done for you by my Father in heaven' (Matthew 18:19). The Greek word for 'agree' used in the verse is the source for our word 'symphony.' Two people praying in agreement make beautiful music to God!"[1]

The apostle Paul understood this dynamic. Although he was one of the most effective Christians who ever lived, he also understood His weaknesses. He depended on his friends. He constantly wrote to them, asking them—even pleading with them—to pray for him. Imitating the pattern of Paul's life of requesting prayer is another way we can give control to Christ. We will take a look at this idea more closely today.

Paul often asked believers to pray for him. Read Romans 15:30-32. What two things does Paul request the believers to ask for in prayer?

_____

_____

_____

Read Ephesians 6:19-20. What two things does Paul request the believers to ask for in prayer?

_____

_____

_____

Read 2 Thessalonians 3:1-2. What two things does Paul request the believers to ask for in prayer?

_____

_____

_____

What similarities do you notice in each of these requests?

_____

_____

_____

Paul made a slightly different request for prayer in his letter to friend Philemon. Read Philemon 1:22. What was Paul's request?

_____

_____

_____

To what degree do you currently ask your friends to pray for you?

_____

_____

_____

When people pray for you and your needs, you allow the Holy Spirit to work in many lives as He ministers to you. The lives of those who pray for you are enriched by connecting with the Lord. God never leaves you alone, and He provides Christian friends to give earthly support to His heavenly ministry. So this week, make sure that you fill out the weekly prayer request form and turn it in when you attend your group meeting. When you draw out a prayer request form, make a special commitment to pray for that person this week. By doing so, you will allow others to be enriched, and your life will be enriched as well!

Lord, thank You for sending people into my life who care about me and pray for me. Father, help me to become a person who shows love and care for others by becoming a true prayer warrior on others' behalf. Amen.

REFLECTION AND APPLICATION

Day 6

Heavenly Father, use me as a vehicle to help others yield their lives to You. Let me be a minister to them and strengthen them in their faith. Amen.

Being part of a small group of a trusted community of believers gives you the perfect opportunity to put into practice the principles you have studied this week. Your Christian friends give you the support and love in times of need, and you return that love and support whenever you pray for a friend, take a meal to them when they are sick, or just sit and listen when they need to talk.

One way to minister to your friends is by sharing a passage in Scripture with them. This is especially effective if you have been through a situation similar to the one they are facing and found that passage to be a source of encouragement during your time of need. Grouping verses into categories that apply to different situations will provide you with appropriate verses that you can use to minister to others. Even if you are not a gifted speaker, sincere words spoken in love give comfort and encouragement to those who need it.

Of course, you need to follow the Holy Spirit's leading when you do this. The Bible says that "all Scripture is God-breathed and is useful for teaching, rebuking, correcting and training in righteousness" (2 Timothy 3:16), but this should be done in love and for the purpose of bringing restoration in the person's life. Speak the truth when you need to do so, but be careful that you are not using it just to judge that person. As Paul wrote, "This is my prayer: that your love may abound more and more in knowledge and depth of insight, so that you may be able to discern what is best and may be pure and blameless until the day of Christ" (Philippians 1:9-10). When you love others, you will want the best for them.

If you haven't already started a notebook, file, or prayer journal for your memory verses, it isn't too late. Any time is a good time to begin memorizing Scripture, and you will discover what a difference those verses can make in your life and ministry.

Father, I have been justified through faith and have peace with You through my Lord Jesus Christ (see Romans 5:1). Thank You for Your mercy. Amen.

Day 7 REFLECTION AND APPLICATION

Lord, You are everything good, everything perfect, everything righteous. Thank You for Your provision. Amen.

Someone once asked Bible teacher Charles Stanley if a person could live by faith and still set goals. Stanley told the person that he would have to think about it. Eventually, he came to the conclusion that yes, a person could live by faith and still set goals, provided the goals were in accordance with God's goals for the person's life.[2]

When you set goals for yourself, where do you go for guidance? David said, "Your word is a lamp to my feet and a light for my path" (Psalm 119:105). Go to the Bible for guidance. Hide God's Word in your heart, and you will always have His light to direct your decisions and actions throughout the day. Start with Scripture, prayerfully asking the Holy Spirit to guide you, and then look at prudence, wisdom and feasibility. In addition, ask trusted Christians to speak into your life and help you decide which way is right and true. Let the peace of God reign in your heart (see Colossians 3:15) as you pray that God would reveal the right way to go.

Think about recent decisions you have made in your life. How has God played a part in those decisions?

_____

_____

_____

_____

Have you ever made a decision you thought God wanted you to make, only to discover He wanted you to go an entirely different way? How can hiding God's Word in your heart help you in the future?

_____

_____

_____

_____

How is memorizing Scripture a valuable weapon in your battle against the evil one? How can it help you overcome any obstacle?

_____

_____

_____

_____

Lord, help me listen to advice from Your Word and to accept instruction so that I will be wise (see Proverbs 19:20).

Notes
1. Elmer Towns, *How to Pray When You Don't Know What to Say* (Ventura, CA: Regal, 2006), p. 82.
2. Charles Stanley, *In Touch with God* (Nashville, TN: Thomas Nelson, 1997), p. 135.

Group Prayer Requests

4 first place
health

Today's Date: _____

Name	Request

Results

_____

_____

_____

_____

_____

_____

a life of
purpose

SCRIPTURE MEMORY VERSE
*May God himself, the God of peace, sanctify you through
and through. May your whole spirit, soul and body be kept
blameless at the coming of our Lord Jesus Christ.*
1 THESSALONIANS 5:23

Ronald Reagan once said, "My philosophy of life is that if we make up
our mind what we are going to make of our lives, then work hard toward
that goal, we never lose." During these last weeks of this study, we've focused on some specific goals for giving Christ control and leading a balanced life. The goals are significant, but what really counts is taking a
long-term approach to health and balance—mentally, physically, emotionally and spiritually. What really matters is being "sanctified," or being set apart so that God can use us to achieve His purposes on earth.

The concept of sanctification can be a bit difficult to grasp, but it
basically means as we consecrate, or set apart, our lives to doing the will
of the Lord, He does a work within our lives through the power of the
Holy Spirit. He gives us the power to follow His plan and focus on His
goals for our lives so that we "might become an offering acceptable to
God, sanctified by the Holy Spirit" (Romans 15:16).

In this week's study, we'll read about the life of the apostle Paul and
how he continually relied on Christ to sanctify him. We will examine
how Paul kept himself blameless for the Lord Jesus Christ. As we look at
his life, you will have an opportunity to think about your own goals and
how they fit into God's plans.

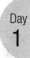
Day
1

LIVING WITH PURPOSE

O Lord Jesus, let me always live to please You. I live by Your grace. Amen.

There's a famous sequence in Lewis Carroll's *Alice's Adventures in Wonderland* that accurately sums up the way that we sometimes chase our goals. In the story, Alice is lost and asks directions from the Cheshire Cat, a feline who has the annoying habit of appearing and disappearing at will. Alice asks the Cat, "Would you tell me, please, which way I ought to go from here?"

"That depends a good deal on where you want to get to," says the Cat.

"I don't much care where—" says Alice.

"Then it doesn't matter which way you go," answers the Cat.

"—so long as I get somewhere," Alice adds as an explanation.

"Oh, you're sure to do that," says the Cat, "if you only walk enough."[1]

What is your purpose in life? It can be easy to slip into a pattern of living—get up, get ready, eat breakfast, go to work, come home, eat dinner, watch TV, go to bed, get up the next day and do it all over again. We sometimes can focus so much on the day-to-day living that we lose track of the greater purpose. We're content to get somewhere, but that's not necessarily the place that God wants us to be.

Some goals describe the destination. Other goals become the map that charts the route between where we are and where we want to be. But God wants us to yield our lives to Him for a reason. What we do fits into His greater design. Part of the adventure in life is discovering that design and sensing the potential that we have in Him. Let's look at this idea more closely today.

Read Philippians 3:7-11. What does Paul say is his primary purpose in life (see vv. 7-8)?

_____

_____

_____

Paul was excited about the things that Christ was doing in him, but his primary focus was in knowing and serving Christ and to be blameless before Him. Take a closer look at the passage in Philippians that you just read, and then complete the phrases below:

I consider everything a _____ compared to the surpassing greatness of knowing Christ Jesus . . . I consider them rubbish, that I may gain Christ and be _____ him. . . . I want to _____ Christ and the _____ of his resurrection and the _____ of _____ his sufferings, becoming like him in his _____, and so, somehow, to attain the _____ from the dead.

How would you describe your life's purpose?

_____

_____

_____

To what degree are you able to say, along with Paul, that knowing Christ and experiencing the things in the phrases you just completed are the most important goals of your life? Explain.

_____

_____

_____

_____

How does the concept of living by grace fit with the idea of living to please God? (Hint: see Romans 8:1-17.)

_____

_____

_____

Read 2 Corinthians 5:9. In the following table, write out the ways that you can apply this verse to your life as it relates to living a balanced life spiritually, emotionally, physically and mentally.

Spiritually	Emotionally
Physically	Mentally

In Micah 6:8 we read, "What does the LORD require of you? To act justly and to love mercy and to walk humbly with your God." What do you think of the simple plan for a purposeful life that is laid out in this verse?

_____

_____

_____

How might your own purpose be similarly simple and straightforward?

_____

_____

_____

Heavenly Father, help me to be blameless before You by knowing You more fully and consistently living to please You. Thank You for Your grace. Amen.

Day 2

RESTING IN THE GOD OF PEACE

Jesus, for Your sake I consider everything a loss compared to the surpassing greatness of knowing You. Help me to live a sanctified life for You. Amen.

It sounds horrible, but sometimes when ancient Roman armies conquered an enemy, soldiers strapped the bodies of the dead onto the backs of the prisoners and forced them to carry the corpses as they decomposed. This practice surely disgusts us today, yet many people still "strap on" metaphoric corpses and carry them around with them. Perhaps these corpses are painful memories of past failures. Or perhaps their current sins have entangled them and are now weighing them down.

Fortunately, in Christ past sins can be forgiven. Past failure can provide motivation for positive future living. To know that we made a mistake in our past provides us with knowledge that we can use to become wiser today. When we accepted Christ as our Savior, He freed us from those past sins and set us apart as children of God. Because of this, we can experience the peace of knowing that we can live a sanctified life for God. Let's look at this idea more closely today.

What do you know about Paul's past life? (Hint: see Galatians 1:13-14.) Describe some of his actions.

_____

_____

_____

_____

Read 1 Corinthians 15:9-10. How does Paul describe his past life?

_____

_____

_____

Read 1 Timothy 1:12-16. According to Paul, why was he shown mercy? What do you think he means by this statement?

_____

_____

_____

How does Paul view Christ's righteous character in light of his sin?

_____

_____

_____

According to Romans 8:6, what is the source of Paul's peace?

_____

_____

_____

Read Ephesians 2:13-15. What does this say about the peace of God?

_____

_____

_____

In what ways have you known God to be a God of peace?

_____

_____

_____

How will focusing on the peace of God help you continually yield your life to Him?

_____

_____

_____

Jesus, You are my peace. It doesn't matter what I have done; You are able and willing to forgive all my sins. Thank You for forgiving me. Because of Your work on the cross, I am whiter than snow. Amen.

Day 3

SET FREE

Lord Jesus, help me continually walk with You. Thank You for setting me free from sin. Let me continually step into my new identity in Christ. Amen.

In *The Pilgrim's Progress*, John Bunyan tells the story of Christian, an everyman character who embarks on a journey from his hometown, the City of Destruction, to the heavenly Celestial City. As the narrative opens, Christian finds himself weighed down by a great burden that he cannot get rid of by himself. He knows that he needs deliverance from this burden, so he goes in search of someone who can help. He speaks to a number of individuals that explain the message of salvation to him and point him to the Place of Deliverance. There, at the foot of the cross, the straps that bind his burden break, and he is free.

As believers, Christ has set us free from the burdens that have weighed us down. We do not have to sin anymore. We have been set free! When we completely give up control of our lives to God and accept His will, He fills our souls with peace and empowers us to live sanctified lives. It's a simple idea, but also a radical one. Let's explore this more closely today.

What does 1 Corinthians 6:17 tell you about the Holy Spirit?

_____

_____

_____

Bible teacher Beth Moore says that the key to victory "is to bow daily . . . to the control of the Holy Spirit over your body."[2] God wants to have control over every part of our being. If we let Him control only one or two parts, we miss the full meaning and joy of His peace. What does Paul say about this peace in Colossians 3:15?

_____

_____

_____

_____

What do you think it means to let God's peace "rule" in your heart? Give some practical examples.

_____

_____

_____

_____

The soul represents the heart of our emotions, feelings and personality. If we let any one part control our lives—such as harmful eating habits, negative attitudes or out-of-control feelings—we distance ourselves from the God of peace. We let our physical appetite and drives take over, and they become the authority by which we live. What good advice does Paul give in Colossians 3:5 about our earthly natures?

_____

_____

_____

What might it look like, practically, to "put to death" whatever belongs to our sinful natures?

_____

_____

_____

Read Colossians 3:12, how are we to clothe ourselves as God's chosen?

_____

_____

_____

What might this look like practically?

_____

_____

_____

When we give Christ control over our lives, we are invited to claim the promise set forth in Philippians 4:6-7: "Do not be anxious about anything, but in everything, by prayer and petition, with thanksgiving, present your requests to God. And the peace of God, which transcends all understanding, will guard your hearts and your minds in Christ Jesus." As you conclude today's study, write some ways that you can apply this verse to your life today.

God, I want to live every minute of my life in Your presence. Help me live to please You always. You are my peace, and I will rest in You. Amen.

FAITHFUL TO THE END

O Lord, let me live my whole life for You. When I reach the end of my days, I want to look back and say that I followed You wholeheartedly. Amen.

After Paul's conversion, his stated goal in life was to know Christ and live to please Him. Paul kept his mind on the goal. More than anything else, he wanted to experience Christ in every part of his being. He understood what Christ had done for him. He remembered his sin for which Christ had died, and he understood the power of Christ's mercy, grace and love. May our goals be the same!

In his letters to the church at Thessalonica, Paul urged the Christians to encourage each other as they served God. In 1 Thessalonians 5:14-18, what specific things did Paul tell them to do? Make a list below.

_____

_____

_____

According to Romans 8:6, what is the reward of one whose mind is controlled by the Spirit?

_____

_____

_____

How can we encourage others to live this way?

_____

_____

_____

Read 1 Corinthians 9:23-27. What things did Paul said he did in order to obtain his goal?

_____

_____

_____

According to this passage, how did Paul define "the prize"?

_____

_____

_____

Read 2 Timothy 4:6-8. What things were important to Paul as he neared the end of his life and ministry?

_____

_____

_____

_____

As you conclude today's study, think about whether you will be able to say something similar to what Paul said at the end of your life and ministry. How will you remember your life when you look back? Paul says that there is a crown of righteousness in store for all who have "longed for [Christ's] appearing." Are you focused on pursuing the prize? If not, what do you need to do in your life to refocus your priorities?

_____

_____

_____

_____

Heavenly Father, help me to be surrendered totally to You. I want to fully surrender control so that You can use my life for Your special service. I bow before You and recognize You as the one true God. Amen.

YEILDING YOURSELF FOR A BIG GOAL

Day 5

O Lord, let me only want what You want for my life. Let me be faithful in the small areas and faithful in the large areas. Amen.

Dr. Henrietta Mears (1890-1963) lived her life with one purpose: to inspire a generation of college students to Christian leadership because of their faith. Billy Graham, Bill Bright and more than four hundred other students became pastors, chaplains, missionaries or inspirational speakers as a result of Dr. Mears's mentoring. In addition to working as the Christian Education director at Hollywood First Presbyterian Church, Dr. Mears also established Forest Home Conference Center, GLINT International and Gospel Light and Regal Books.

Dr. Mears recognized the benefit of starting small and humbling herself before the Lord so that He could lift her up in His timing (see James 4:10). But she also recognized the value of pursuing huge dreams. She recognized the value of seasons of preparation, yet for her there was always a greater goal of influencing others for Christ—and as many people as possible. For her, only an amazing life for Christ would do.

She wrote, "So many people are willing to be bellhops for the Lord, standing around waiting for someone to give them some little errand to do for Him, instead of asking the Lord to give them His greatest will for their lives. There are so few who want to do the big things for God. You should not be content to pump the organ if God wants you to play on it."[3]

Today, we will look at the Bible's "Hall of Faith" in Hebrews 11 and see how each of these biblical figures remained true to the larger goal.

Read Hebrews 11:8-28. List some of the "large" accomplishments of the people mentioned here.

_____

_____

_____

_____

_____

According to this passage, what was the one key element in each of these people's lives?

_____

_____

_____

When you personally think about doing something large or great for Christ, what dreams come to mind?

_____

_____

_____

What can you do in your daily life to keep yourself ready for His service?

_____

_____

_____

Sometimes living a life of faith means enduring hardships. During Paul's ministry, he endured many hardships, such as imprisonment, floggings, beatings, stonings and shipwrecks (see 2 Corinthians 11:23-29). However, God offers us some incredible encouragement to persevere. Read through the verses in the following table, and then summarize the encouragement contained in each one in the right-hand column.

Verse	Encouragement
Joshua 1:9	
Psalm 46:1	
Isaiah 41:10	

Verse	Encouragement
Romans 8:38-39	
Hebrews 13:5	
1 John 4:4	

Today, say a prayer of thanksgiving to God that whatever we face in this life, we have the assurance that He will always be with us.

Thank You, Father, for being faithful to Your Word and for giving me Your peace. I place my life in Your hands. Amen.

REFLECTION AND APPLICATION

My prayer, dear Lord, is that You would help me to give control of my life to You. You are good, and I know I have nothing to fear. Amen.

The Bible doesn't tell us how Paul ultimately ended his journey on this earth. We know that he was arrested in Jerusalem around AD 57 and held as a prisoner for two years. Then, in AD 59, he appealed to Caesar as was his right as a Roman citizen and was sent to Rome for a trial. After enduring a shipwreck on Malta, he arrived in Rome in AD 60 and spent two more years under house arrest. The last verse in Acts states that there he "boldly and without hindrance . . . preached the kingdom of God and taught about the Lord Jesus Christ" (Acts 28:31).

Perhaps that is the best place to end his story. For whatever the truth, Paul's fate was secondary to that of the gospel. Luke's final picture of Paul shows him doing what he has done throughout the book of Acts: preaching the message of Christ. Despite the hardships he endured, he refused to stop sharing the love of Christ with everyone he met.

As the first-century Church father Clement wrote, "Paul by his example pointed out the prize of patient endurance . . . he won the noble renown which was the reward of his faith, having taught righteousness unto the whole world and having reached the farthest bounds of the West; and when he had borne his testimony before the rulers, so he departed from the world and went unto the holy place, having been found a notable pattern of patient endurance."

As we strive to honor the Lord by living balanced lives, we know we will face obstacles and need to overcome strongholds. Yet no matter what the challenge, we know that we have weapons of divine power for our use (see Ephesians 6:10-18). Prayer and the Word of God are two of our most powerful weapons to help us stay on track. So let's do some praying right now. Ask the Lord to help you continually yield control of your life to Him. You may want to use the following prompts below.

Lord God, help me continually be joyful in hope, patient in affliction and faithful in prayer (see Romans 12:11-12). Thank You, Lord God. Amen.

Father God, I thank You for everything that was written in the past to teach me so that through endurance and the encouragement of the Scriptures I might have hope (see Romans 15:4). Amen.

Gracious Father, I thank You for giving me weapons that have the divine power to demolish strongholds (see 2 Corinthians 10:4). Amen.

Day 7

REFLECTION AND APPLICATION

Oh Lord God, You are truly gracious. Thank You that I am Your child. You are truly good, and I worship You. Amen.

As you come to the end of this study, you may be evaluating your goals and what ways your life has become more balanced during these past weeks. How do you measure your success? Is it strictly by pounds lost, or are you seeing the overall picture of growing more to be like Christ? Today, simply allow the Lord to encourage you. Read the passages below and rest in the knowledge of your identity in Christ. Use the blank spaces below to journal any thoughts you have or prayers to the Lord after each statement.

You are a child of God. "Yet to all who received him, to those who believed in his name, he gave the right to become children of God" (John 1:12).

_____

_____

_____

You are free from condemnation. "Therefore, there is now no condemnation for those who are in Christ Jesus" (Romans 8:1).

_____

_____

_____

You are complete in Christ. "You have been given fullness in Christ, who is the head over every power and authority" (Colossians 2:10).

_____

_____

_____

You can do all things through Christ. "I can do everything through him who gives me strength" (Philippians 4:13).

_____

_____

_____

Notes

1. Lewis Caroll, *Alice's Adventures in Wonderland* (New York: Signet Classics, 2000).
2. Beth Moore, *Praying God's Word* (Nashville, TN: B&H, 2000), p. 150.
3. Barbara Hudson, *The Henrietta Mears Story* (Grand Rapids, MI: Revell, 1957), p. 166.

Group Prayer Requests

4 first place health

Today's Date: _____

Name	Request

Results

_____

_____

_____

_____

_____

_____

time to celebrate!

To help shape your brief victory celebration testimony, work through the following questions in your prayer journal:

Day One: List some of the benefits you have gained by allowing the Lord to transform your life through this 12-week First Place 4 Health session. Be sure to list benefits you have received in the physical, mental, emotional and spiritual realms of your being.

Day Two: In what ways have you most significantly changed *mentally*? Have you seen a shift in the ways you think about yourself, food, your relationships or God? How has Scripture memory been a part of these shifts?

Day Three: In what ways have you most significantly changed *emotionally*? Have you begun to identify how your feelings influence your relationship to food and exercise? What are you doing to stay aware of your emotions, both positive and negative?

Day Four: In what ways have you most significantly changed *spiritually*? How has your relationship with God deepened? How has drawing closer to Him made a difference in the other three areas of your life?

Day Five: In what ways have you most significantly changed *physically*? Have you met or exceeded your weight/measurement goals? How has your health improved the past 12 weeks?

Day Six: Was there one person in your First Place 4 Health group who was particularly encouraging to you? How did their kindness make a difference in your First Place 4 Health journey?

Day Seven: Summarize the previous six questions into a one-page testimony, or "faith story," to share at your group's victory celebration.

May our gracious Lord bless and keep you as you continue to keep Him first in all things!

Giving Christ Control
leader discussion guide

For in-depth information, guidance and helpful tips about leading a successful First Place 4 Health group, study the *First Place 4 Health Leader's Guide*. In it, you will find valuable answers to most of your questions, as well as personal insights from many First Place 4 Health group leaders.

For the group meetings in this session, be sure to read and consider each week's discussion topics several days before the meeting—some questions and activities require supplies and/or planning to complete. Also, if you are leading a large group, plan to break into smaller groups for discussion and then come together as a large group to share your answers and responses. Make sure to appoint a capable leader for each small group so that discussions stay focused and on track (and be sure each group records their answers!).

week one: welcome to *Giving Christ Control*

During this first week, welcome the members to your group, provide a brief overview of the First Place 4 Health program, explain what is expected of the participants at each of the weekly meetings, and collect the Member Surveys. (See the *First Place 4 Health Leader's Guide* for a detailed outline of how to conduct the first week's meeting.)

week two: relying on His goodness

In this week's study, members looked at how they can always rely on God's goodness during the good times, the bad times and all the uncertain times in between. Start today's lesson by asking members to consider the phrase "God is good." How is this both a simple and a complex fact as it relates to their lives?

Throughout the story of creation in Genesis 1:4-18, we see the phrase "and God saw that it was good" repeated several times. Ask members what this implies about the nature of God and how the knowledge of God's goodness can help them rest in Him.

On Day Two, participants were asked to consider the best thing that has happened in their lives recently. Have the group share their responses. Discuss how that experience was a reflection of the goodness of God.

The reading for this day's study was in John 2:1-11. The members were asked to describe what they pictured a typical Jewish wedding would be like. Have them share their answers, and then discuss what it says about the character of Christ to know that He celebrated at a wedding.

Have the group members share one thing that has happened recently to them (or that they are still going through) in which the way seemed particularly unclear and uncertain.

Discuss the fact that even though Peter had the faith to step out of the boat—proof that he was moving in the will of Jesus—he quickly began to doubt. Ask the participants if they have ever questioned God's will when they have stepped into His promises for their lives.

On Day Four, members were asked to read Psalm 23. Discuss how many times we want God to lead us by green pastures and cool waters, but we ignore the fact that He also leads us through valleys and shadowy times.

Have someone read Romans 8:28. Ask members how this verse might (or might not) relate to their lives. What does Paul tell us in this verse that we can know even when things don't turn out the way we hoped?

Ask the group members if they have ever thought of themselves as filled with God's goodness. Why or why not?

Have someone read Philippians 2:13 aloud to the group. Discuss how God works in us to "will and to act according to his good purpose" and what this looks like in our everyday lives.

week three: convinced of His love

Giving control of our lives to God is much easier when we remember that God loves us and always has our best interests at heart. God is favorably inclined toward us, so we can have the confidence that if we place ourselves in His hands, He will take care of us. Ask participants to discuss the phrase "God is love." What does this—or doesn't this—mean?

In his first letter, John discusses God's love a great deal and explains how we should share that love with others. Have someone read 1 John 4:8. What are the implications of this verse?

The single greatest extended biblical definition of love is found in 1 Corinthians 13:1-12, which members read during the Day Two study. Discuss some of the gifts and "good deeds" Paul lists in verses 1-3 and what he says about the value of these things if we do not have the love of God.

Writing down a descriptive word can help us to remember the extent of Christ's love for us. Ask the group members to share the word they came up with during the study. Why did they choose that particular word?

Perhaps the best-known parable about God's love is the story of the prodigal son in Luke 11:15-32. Ask someone to summarize the story. Discuss what the father's actions reveal about his love for his wayward son.

On Day Four, members read Psalm 131, a short psalm depicting God's love. Ask the group to describe the imagery used in this psalm and some of the practical applications they wrote out based on these verses.

"In times of trial or difficulty, our invitation is to press in closer to the Lord." Ask the group members what they think about when they read this statement. How can hardships be part of God's plan for our lives? In what ways do they make us draw closer to the Lord?

Ask the members how knowing that God asks them to let Him carry their burdens prompts them to yield their lives more completely to Him.

Close in prayer, thanking God for His gift of grace and His incredible love for each of us.

week four: yielding to His glory

Begin the discussion time by asking the members to give their reflections on how the glory of the Lord is described in Psalm 19:1-6.

During the Day One study, participants read in Hebrews 12:1-3 that we are to "fix our eyes on Jesus." Discuss what that means and have the group members provide some practical examples of how we can do this.

Have someone read 2 Corinthians 10:5, and then discuss what it means to "take captive every thought and make it obedient to Christ."

Members were asked to consider in what ways they have seen the battle for their minds as a spiritual struggle. Discuss the responses.

God has given each of us powerful weapons to use in this spiritual battle. Have the participants discuss the strategies for warfare and the specific pieces of armor they discovered in their study of Ephesians 6:10-19.

Have someone in the group read Psalm 84:1-2. Ask the members to give their responses to how the psalmist describes the dwelling place of God.

Ask members to discuss the insights they discovered in reading Hebrews 2:18–3:1. How are they encouraged in knowing that Jesus faced the same temptations that we face?

On Day Seven, group members were asked to think about Christ and what is pleasing to Him. Have members share their thoughts when asked what they pictured when they thought of Christ's beauty and majesty and what is true, noble, righteous, pure, admirable, excellent and lovely.

Conclude today's discussion time in prayer, asking God to continue His work in renewing their heart and minds.

week five: control: whose responsibility is it?

God equips each of us to be responsible for our actions while, at the same time, giving control of our lives over to Him. This sounds paradoxical, but self-control and being controlled by Christ always go hand in hand. Have group members discuss how this plays out in their lives.

Have someone in the group read Romans 6:11-13 out loud. Discuss the three principles that Paul explains in this passage.

On Day Three, group members examined five additional principles in 1 Corinthians 10:1-13 to help fight the battle against temptation. Discuss each of these principles and what they look like in our lives.

Have one member in the group read Colossians 1:10 and another read Ephesians 4:1. Have the group discuss what their true motivation for giving Christ control of their lives should be based on these verses.

On Day Four, participants were asked to look up several verses related to God's power in their lives (Romans 4:20-21; Ephesians 3:16-21; 6:10; 2 Timothy 1:7; Colossians 1:29; 2 Peter 1:3) and write the central idea as it relates to their Christian life. Have one person (or two people, depending on time) share their answers for each verse.

Evangelists such as Billy Graham understand the need to set up clear boundaries to avoid even the slightest hint of impropriety. Discuss how boundaries are useful and necessary for leading a balanced life.

Ask participants (who are willing) to share how a careless action they did in the past had a negative impact on another person. What would they have done different?

Discuss what biblical accountability means and why it is beneficial for a Christian to be accountable to a trusted group of believers.

Conclude in prayer, asking the Lord to help members establish clear boundaries so they can resist temptation when it comes their way.

week six: yielding our desires

Begin today's session by having members discuss a few of the things in their lives for which they are thankful and content.

A.W. Tozer once said, "God may allow His servant to succeed when He has disciplined him to a point where he does not need to succeed to be happy." Discuss how true contentment is a life lived fully in God's hands.

On Day One, members were asked to read Philippians 4:10-13. Have someone read this passage again to the group and then discuss what was Paul's secret of "being content in any and every situation."

"Lust" means having out-of-control desires. For instance, if we lust after food, we don't give thought to the consequences of the amount of food we are putting in our bodies. Ask the participants to discuss some of the practical ways they found during the Day Two study for avoiding "lust."

Participants read the parable of the rich fool found in Luke 12:18-21 on Day Three. Discuss what the rich man's mistake was in tearing down his barns to build more. How do his actions demonstrate he had greed in his heart? What in the parable specifically points to this fact?

During the Day Four study, participants read a passage in James addressing the issue of envy. Discuss the source of envy according to James and some of the harmful results it produces.

"Because we have been given new life in Christ, there is nothing that can hold us as spiritual hostages." Ask the group members if they agree with this statement. Why or why not?

Conclude by re-reading this week's memory verse (Philippians 4:12-13). Discuss how we can learn to be content in every situation because we can do everything through Christ Jesus who gives us strength.

week seven: releasing our calling

On Day One, members read passages in Genesis on the story of Joseph. Discuss what Joseph did in his earlier years that could be described as mistakes, lapses in judgment, or ambition.

Even at his lowest point—in an Egyptian prison—Joseph could sense the kindness and favor of the Lord. Ask participants to share how they have seen God's presence at work in their lives during their lowest times.

At the end of the story of Joseph, he could realize that the events of his life had happened for a great purpose. Ask the participants what similar confidence they can have that God will work all things for His good.

On Day Two, members examined how they should release their "destinations" to God. Ask participants if they've ever hoped the Lord would guide them to a specific location or position. If so, what was it?

Discuss the three things Abram was asked to leave behind and what God promised to him if he obeyed.

On Day Three, the members looked at releasing their security to God. Discuss what sorts of things in their lives are within their control and what things are beyond their control. How does that make them feel when they consider this reality?

Discuss how Gideon on three separate occasions asked for God to give him the security in knowing that He was truly with him.

Finances are a regular concern for many people. On Day Four, members were asked to take a look at their attitudes about money and some of what the Bible teaches about money. Ask them what they discovered.

Discuss what members discovered during the Day Five study about how they can release their pasts to Christ and move forward in His plan.

week eight: surrendering our words

Begin with a discussion of how the members have seen the power of words in their lives—whether for good or ill—and how they can give control of those words to the Lord.

During the Day One study, members read the story of Nabal. Discuss what the situation was that made David so angry at Nabal's response and what the consequences of those misspoken words were for Nabal.

On Day Two, participants took a test on how well they controlled their words. Have those who are willing share their results with the group and what they discovered from the exercise.

Have someone in the group read James 3:9. Ask the group why they think it is so important to guard our words and what the consequences can be if we do not.

Two types of negative speech are gossip and slander. Ask the participants what they discovered during their Day Three study about the seriousness of these types of speech.

On Day Four, members were asked to write their own versions of Psalm 136 using the repeated line "His love endures forever." Ask those who are willing to share their findings.

On Day Five, participants looked at how what they say can be a vehicle to bring healing to others. Ask the group to discuss the passages they looked up that would enable them to help and heal others (Ephesians 1:15-16; Colossians 3:13,16; 1 Thessalonians 5:11,14; 1 Peter 2:17) and share what they discovered.

Conclude today's study in prayer, thanking God that He gives each of us the ability to bring healing into other people's lives.

week nine: how to let go of control

Ask someone to read Luke 9:23 and discuss the three commitments Jesus said are a part of following Him. What are some of the most challenging aspects in following these commitments and living a balanced life?

Ask the members what they like to do that actively demonstrates Christ's love to others. How could they view these activities as their "ministry"?

Ask the group what it means to abide in Christ. What sorts of things do they do to connect with the Lord on a daily basis?

Ask members to discuss the habits and heart attitudes they have developed that enables them to stay close to the Lord. Is there anything they would like to change about their quiet time with the Lord?

Have someone in the group read John 15:7. Discuss the two conditions that Jesus gives for the promise in this passage to be fulfilled.

Ask those in the group to reflect on how they typically view prayer. Do they feel it is a duty or discipline, or something they enjoy doing? How is prayer like having a conversation with a loved one?

Discuss what was unique about how the early believers interacted with each other.

Ask the group members to discuss some of their feelings and hang-ups when they picture themselves doing evangelism.

week ten: a community of encouragement

Swiss physician Paul Tournier once said, "There are two things we cannot do alone. One is to be married, and the other is to be a Christian." Ask participants if they agree or disagree with this statement, and why.

During the Day One study, members looked at how the apostle Paul conducted his relationships with those in the Thessalonian church. Discuss how Paul described his role as a spiritual father.

Ask the members if they have ever been part of a group in which a spiritual mother or father responded to them the way that Paul did with his friends. What would it take to have such relationships in a group?

On Day Two, members read about a crisis situation in the church in Jerusalem. Discuss what brought about this crisis and how the church in Antioch responded to the need. How was Barnabas an encourager?

Discuss some practical ways that each group member can encourage those in his or her life.

"Blind spots" are areas we cannot see clearly and must always check. Ask the members if there has been a time when a trusted friend helped them with a blind spot, or if they've ever helped a friend in this area.

On Day Three, participants looked at Jesus' words in Matthew 7:1-5. Discuss how taking the time to remove the plank from our own eye prepares us to help with the speck in another person's eye.

Ask participants if they've ever experienced the concept of spiritual "stuckness." What happened, and how did they get going again?

Discuss how the writer of Hebrews says that we are supposed to help others stay out of such spiritual loops (see Hebrews 3:12-13).

Discuss to what degree members currently ask their friends to pray for them. Conclude today's study by breaking up into groups of one to three people and having the members pray for each other.

week eleven: a life of purpose

Begin this week's session by sharing this quote from Oliver Wendell Holmes: "The greatest thing in this world is not so much where we are, but in what direction we're moving." Ask participants if they agree or disagree with the saying, and why.

On Day One, members looked at what Paul said was his primary purpose in Philippians 3:7-11. Discuss what this purpose was. How would the participants currently define their life's purpose?

In Day Two, the group members examined how they can rest in the peace of God. Discuss what it means to truly rest in the peace that Christ brings. In what ways have the members experienced the peace of God?

Ask someone to read Colossians 3:15. Discuss what it means to allow God's peace to rule in our hearts. Ask for some practical examples.

Paul urged the Christians in Thessalonica to encourage each other as they served God. Discuss what Paul told them to do in 1 Thessalonians 5:14-18 to do. (Participants were asked to make a list, so have them share what they found.)

During the Day Five study, members examined some of the characters listed in the Bible's "Hall of Faith" in Hebrews 11. Have participants list some of the "large" accomplishments of the people mentioned there. What was the one key element present in each of these people's lives?

Discuss the things that Paul did while pursuing his goal (see 1 Corinthians 9:23-27). How did Paul define "the prize"?

As you conclude today's session, remind group members that they will be sharing their testimonies as part of next week's victory celebration. Conclude in prayer, thanking God for the purpose that He gives to every person's life.

week twelve: time to celebrate!

Even though most of your meeting this week will be a victory celebration, take some time at the beginning of the meeting to talk about how much God loves each person in the group and how each of us is called to yield the control of our lives to Him. (See "Planning a Victory Celebration" in the *First Place 4 Health Leader's Guide* for ideas about throwing a successful celebration for your group.)

For the rest of the study time, allow each member to tell his or her *Giving Christ Control* story. Give members an equal opportunity to share the goals they set for themselves at the beginning of the session and talk about the challenges and good things God has done for them throughout the process. Don't allow the more talkative group members to monopolize all the time. Even the quiet members need an opportunity to share their stories and successes! Even those who have not met their goals have still been part of the journey, so allow them to share and talk about why they did not succeed.

Making a commitment to continue in First Place 4 Health is an important part of encouraging people in their quest to yield their lives to Christ. Be sure to talk about your group's future plans, and make each person feel welcome to continue to journey with you.

First Place 4 Health
menu plans

Each menu plan is based on approximately 1,400 to 1,500 calories per day. All recipe and menu exchanges were determined using the Master-Cook software, a program that accesses a database containing more than 6,000 food items prepared using the United States Department of Agriculture (USDA) publications and information from food manu-facturers. As with any nutritional program, MasterCook calculates the nutritional values of the recipes based on ingredients. Nutrition may vary due to how the food is prepared, where the food comes from, soil content, season, ripeness, processing and method of preparation. For these reasons, please use the recipes and menu plans as approximate guides. Consult a physician and/or a registered dietitian before start-ing a weight-loss program.

For those who need more calories, add the following to the 1,400-calorie plan:

- 1,800 calories: 2 ounce equivalent of meat, 3 ounce equivalent of bread, $^1/_2$ cup vegetable serving, 1 tsp. fat

- 2,000 calories: 2 ounce equivalent of meat, 4 ounce equivalent of bread, $^1/_2$ cup vegetable serving, 3 tsp. fat

- 2,200 calories: 2 ounce equivalent of meat, 5 ounce equivalent of bread, $^1/_2$ cup vegetable serving, $^1/_2$ cup fruit serving, 5 tsp. fat

- 2,400 calories: 2 ounce equivalent of meat, 6 ounce equivalent of bread, 1 cup vegetable serving, $^1/_2$ cup fruit serving, 6 tsp. fat

First Week Grocery List

Produce
- ❑ apples (Red Delicious and Granny Smith)
- ❑ asparagus
- ❑ bananas
- ❑ broccoli
- ❑ cabbage, finely shredded (1 pkg.)
- ❑ cantaloupe
- ❑ carrots
- ❑ celery
- ❑ garlic cloves
- ❑ grapefruit
- ❑ honeydew melon
- ❑ lemons
- ❑ lettuce
- ❑ mushrooms
- ❑ onions
- ❑ oranges
- ❑ peaches
- ❑ pears
- ❑ potatoes
- ❑ red grapes
- ❑ red onions
- ❑ red potatoes
- ❑ romaine lettuce
- ❑ spinach
- ❑ strawberries
- ❑ tomatoes
- ❑ watermelon
- ❑ zucchini

Baking Products
- ❑ all-fruit spread
- ❑ applesauce, unsweetened
- ❑ black pepper
- ❑ brown sugar
- ❑ canola oil
- ❑ chili powder
- ❑ cumin, ground
- ❑ Dijon mustard
- ❑ dill, dried
- ❑ granulated garlic
- ❑ instant chicken bouillon
- ❑ lemon juice
- ❑ light salad dressing
- ❑ lime juice
- ❑ mustard
- ❑ nonstick cooking spray
- ❑ onion powder
- ❑ onion ranch-style dressing mix
- ❑ paprika
- ❑ peanut butter
- ❑ poultry seasoning
- ❑ raisins
- ❑ ranch dressing, reduced-fat
- ❑ salsa
- ❑ salt
- ❑ soy sauce
- ❑ Sweet'N Low® sweetener
- ❑ sweet pickle relish
- ❑ sugar
- ❑ walnuts

Breads and Cereals
- ❑ blueberry muffin, reduced-fat
- ❑ bread, whole-wheat
- ❑ breadsticks
- ❑ brown rice
- ❑ Cheerios® cereal
- ❑ cornflake crumbs
- ❑ dinner rolls
- ❑ English muffins

❑ flour tortillas, reduced-fat
❑ Grape Nuts® cereal
❑ hamburger buns, whole-wheat
❑ instant oatmeal
❑ linguini
❑ Mexican rice
❑ pita bread, fat-free whole-wheat
❑ Rice Chex® cereal

Canned Foods
❑ chicken broth
❑ 28 oz. Italian-style tomatoes, diced (1 can)
❑ 11 oz. Mexican-style corn (1 can)
❑ pear halves in juice (1 can)
❑ refried beans, reduced-fat

Dairy Products
❑ cheddar cheese, reduced-fat
❑ cottage cheese, 2-percent
❑ eggs
❑ margarine, light
❑ mayonnaise, light
❑ milk, skim
❑ Monterrey Jack cheese
❑ Mozzarella cheese, part-skim

❑ Parmesan cheese
❑ sour cream, reduced-fat
❑ whipped topping, nondairy
❑ yogurt, fruit-flavored nonfat and artificially sweetened
❑ yogurt, pineapple-flavored non-fat and artificially sweetened

Frozen Foods
❑ Stouffer's Frozen Lean Cuisine Entrée®
❑ waffles, whole-wheat

Meat & Poultry
❑ $1^1/_4$ lbs. bay scallops
❑ (4) chicken breasts, boneless and skinless (3 oz. each)
❑ (4) chicken breasts, skinless (4 oz. each)
❑ 1 lb. fish fillets (snapper, tilapia or catfish)
❑ 1 lb. ground round, lean
❑ 1 oz. ham, lean
❑ 1 lb. sirloin steak
❑ turkey bacon
❑ 2 oz. turkey sausage
❑ tuna

First Week Meals and Recipes

DAY 1

....

Breakfast

Turkey Bacon and Egg Sandwich

2 slices whole-wheat bread, toasted

1 egg, cooked in a nonstick pan and
1 strip turkey bacon, cooked crisp

Assemble sandwich and serve with 1 apple. Serves 1.

Nutritional Information: 327 calories; 11g fat (27.7% calories from fat); 14g protein; 47g carbohydrate; 8g dietary fiber; 224mg cholesterol; 549mg sodium.

....

Lunch

Tuna Pocket Sandwich

(1) 7-inch pita bread, whole-wheat
and fat-free
$1/_2$ cup romaine lettuce

$1/_2$ cup tuna
1 tbsp. light mayonnaise
1 tsp. sweet pickle relish

In a small bowl, combine tuna, mayonnaise and pickle relish. Cut pita in half and stuff lettuce and tuna salad inside each half. Serve with $1/_2$ cup carrot sticks, 1 teaspoon reduced-calorie ranch dressing and $1^1/_4$ cups watermelon. Serves 1.

Nutritional Information: 356 calories; 9g fat (21.9% calories from fat); 34g protein; 36g carbohydrate; 4g dietary fiber; 50mg cholesterol; 294mg sodium.

....

Dinner

Oven Fried Chicken

1 cup cornflake crumbs
1 tsp. paprika
1 tsp. instant chicken bouillon
$1/_2$ tsp. poultry seasoning
$1/_2$ cup all-purpose breading mix

$1/_4$ tsp. granulated garlic
$1/_4$ tsp. onion powder
$1/_8$ tsp. black pepper
(4) 4-oz. skinless chicken breasts
nonstick cooking spray

Combine conflake crumbs, paprika, chicken bouillon, poultry seasoning, garlic, onion powder and black pepper to make a breading mix. Mix well and place in an airtight container. (Plan on using 2 tablespoons for each chicken breast.) Preheat oven to 425°F. Place breading in a shallow pan. Spray each breast with the cooking spray and coat each side with the breading mixture. Arrange pieces in a 9" x 9" baking dish that has been coated with cooking spray. Bake for 15 to 20 minutes. Serve each with 1 cup *Coleslaw with Apple* (see recipe below) and a 3-ounce baked potato with 1 teaspoon reduced-fat margarine and 1 teaspoon reduced-fat sour cream. Serves 4.

Coleslaw with Apple

8 oz. finely shredded cabbage
1 small Red Delicious apple, cored
  and finely chopped
1/2 cup fat-free sour cream and
  onion ranch-style dressing mix

1/3 cup thinly sliced celery
2 tsp. lemon juice
1 tsp. sugar

Combine cabbage, apple, and celery in a large bowl. Combine dressing, sugar, and lemon juice in a small bowl, stirring well. Pour dressing mixture over cabbage mixture, and toss well. Cover and chill at least 1 hour. Serves 4.

Nutritional Information: 428 calories; 6g fat (13.4% calories from fat); 40g protein; 51g carbohydrate; 6g dietary fiber; 74mg cholesterol; 778mg sodium.

DAY 2

Breakfast

2 whole-wheat frozen waffles
1/2 cup unsweetened applesauce
1 pkg. Sweet'N Low®

2 tbsp. raisins
1 cup skim milk

Nutritional Information: 372 calories; 6g fat (14.3% calories from fat); 13g protein; 68g carbohydrate; 4g dietary fiber; 27mg cholesterol; 658mg sodium.

Lunch

1 Arby's Regular Roast Beef Sandwich®
1/2 cup celery sticks

3 tbsp. reduced-fat ranch dressing
1 apple

Nutritional Information: 584 calories; 27g fat (41.4% calories from fat); 26g protein; 61g carbohydrate; 9g dietary fiber; 43mg cholesterol; 1,860mg sodium.

Dinner

Beef Stir-Fry

1 pound sirloin steak	1 cup fresh broccoli
1 tsp. chopped garlic	1 cup sliced mushrooms
2 tsp. canola oil	1 tsp. soy sauce
1 red onion	3 tbsp. water
1 cup carrots	4 oz. linguini
1 cup zucchini	nonstick cooking spray

Spray a skillet with cooking spray. Add canola oil and heat over high heat. Add beef and stir-fry with garlic until cooked to your liking. Remove and keep warm. Cook noodles according to package directions. Drain and keep warm. Stir-fry onions and carrots until carrots are partially done; add water as needed to prevent sticking. Add zucchini, broccoli, mushrooms and soy sauce and stir-fry until vegetables are cooked to your liking. Serve with a small breadstick and 1 cup sliced strawberries topped with 1 tablespoon non-dairy whipped topping. Serves 4.

Nutritional Information: 470 calories; 20g fat (35.9% calories from fat); 28g protein; 51g carbohydrate; 7g dietary fiber; 71mg cholesterol; 216mg sodium.

DAY 3

Breakfast

1 pkg. instant oatmeal	1/2 banana, medium-sized
3 walnut halves, chopped	1 cup skim milk

Nutritional Information: 486 calories; 10g fat (18.2% calories from fat); 23g protein; 78g carbohydrate; 11g dietary fiber; 4mg cholesterol; 945mg sodium.

Lunch

Ham Muffin

1 English muffin	1 tomato
1 oz. sliced lean ham	1 tsp. light mayonnaise
lettuce	1/2 tsp. mustard

Assemble muffin and serve with 1 cup broccoli florets with light dressing and pear halves (canned in their own juice) filled with 1/4 cup 2-percent cottage cheese. Serves 1.

Nutritional Information: 381 calories; 5g fat (11.8% calories from fat); 21g protein; 65g carbohydrate; 8g dietary fiber; 20mg cholesterol; 994mg sodium.

Dinner

Scallops Parmesan

1¹/₄ lb. bay scallops	2 tbsp. lemon juice
2 tbsp. light margarine	¹/₄ cup Parmesan cheese,
(1) 28-oz. can diced Italian-style	shredded
tomatoes (not drained)	
1 clove garlic, chopped	

Melt margarine in a skillet over medium-high heat. Sauté garlic and scallops for 3 to 4 minutes, and then add lemon juice and stir. Set aside and keep warm. In a separate skillet, cook tomatoes for 5 to 10 minutes until slightly reduced. Add scallops to tomatoes and heat throughout. Top with Parmesan cheese. Serve with ¹/₂ cup brown rice, 1 cup steamed broccoli and 1 dinner roll. Serves 4.

Nutritional Information: 705 calories; 10g fat (13.4% calories from fat); 42g protein; 110g carbohydrate; 10g dietary fiber; 51mg cholesterol; 1,018mg sodium.

DAY 4

Breakfast

1 medium reduced-fat	1 cup fruit-flavored yogurt, nonfat
blueberry muffin	and artificially sweetened
1 medium peach	

Nutritional Information: 326 calories; 7g fat (18.8% calories from fat); 15g protein; 53g carbohydrate; 5g dietary fiber; 25mg cholesterol; 398mg sodium.

Lunch

Stouffer's Lean Cuisine Entrée®	1 cup fresh citrus sections
Green salad with light dressing	

Nutritional Information: 338 calories; 6g fat (16% calories from fat); 14g protein; 61g carbohydrate; 9g dietary fiber; 40mg cholesterol; 647mg sodium.

Dinner

Salsa Chicken

(4) 3-oz. boneless, skinless
  chicken breasts
2 tbsp. Dijon mustard

2 tsp. brown sugar
2 cups chunky salsa
nonstick cooking spray

Preheat oven to 350°F. Cut each chicken breast into four strips. Arrange pieces in a 9" x 9" baking dish that has been coated with cooking spray. Place chicken in dish and bake uncovered for 10 minutes. Combine remaining ingredients in a small dish and mix until well blended. Flip each strip and pour sauce over chicken and bake an additional 8 to 10 minutes or until chicken is done. Serve with 1/2 cup Mexican rice, 1/2 cup reduced-fat refried beans topped with 2 tablespoons part-skim Mozzarella cheese, shredded lettuce, diced tomatoes, 2 tablespoons reduced-fat sour cream and one reduced-fat 7-inch flour tortilla. Serves 4.

Nutritional Information: 547 calories; 10g fat (16.6% calories from fat); 36g protein; 83g carbohydrate; 9g dietary fiber; 65mg cholesterol; 1,675mg sodium.

DAY 5

Breakfast

3/4 cup Rice Chex® cereal
1/2 English muffin
1 tsp. all-fruit spread

1 cup skim milk
1/2 banana

Nutritional Information: 373 calories; 2g fat (3.8% calories from fat); 13g protein; 78g carbohydrate; 4g dietary fiber; 4mg cholesterol; 468mg sodium.

Lunch

Peanut Butter & Banana Sandwich

2 slices whole-wheat bread
1 1/2 tbsp. peanut butter

1/2 banana, sliced

Serve with 1 cup celery sticks with 1 teaspoon light ranch dressing and 1 medium pear.

Nutritional Information: 455 calories; 16g fat (29.1% calories from fat); 14g protein; 74g carbohydrate; 13g dietary fiber; trace cholesterol; 523mg sodium.

Dinner

Lemon Fish

1 lb. fish fillets (snapper, tilapia or catfish)	2 tsp. light margarine
$^1/_8$ tsp. black pepper	$^1/_4$ cup chicken broth
4 lemon slices	$^1/_8$ tsp. paprika
2 tsp. lemon juice	$^1/_8$ tsp. dried dill

Arrange fish in a 9″ x 13″ baking dish. Top with remaining ingredients in order. Preheat oven to 450°F and bake uncovered for 10 minutes per inch of thickness or until fish flakes easily. Serve with $^3/_4$ cup boiled red potatoes, spinach salad with light dressing, $^1/_2$ cup steamed asparagus with 1 teaspoon melted margarine, and 1 dinner roll. Serves 4.

Nutritional Information: 333 calories; 6g fat (16.3% calories from fat); 29g protein; 42g carbohydrate; 6g dietary fiber; 49mg cholesterol; 382mg sodium.

DAY 6

Breakfast

$^1/_4$ small cantaloupe or honeydew, topped with 1 cup pineapple-flavored yogurt, nonfat and artificially sweetened	$^1/_2$ cup Grape Nuts® cereal, sprinkled on yogurt

Nutritional Information: 311 calories; 2g fat (4.3% calories from fat); 15g protein; 65g carbohydrate; 7g dietary fiber; 3mg cholesterol; 301mg sodium.

Lunch

(1) 6-inch Subway Club Sandwich®	1 cup carrot sticks
2 tbsp. light ranch dressing	15 red grapes

Note: The sandwich should be made with turkey or ham and contain no added fat or cheese (but lots of veggies).

Nutritional Information: 433 calories; 6g fat (11.2% calories from fat); 22g protein; 83g carbohydrate; 10g dietary fiber; 25mg cholesterol; 1,304mg sodium.

Dinner

Tex-Mex Burgers

1 lb. lean ground round
2 tbsp. chili powder
6 whole-wheat hamburger buns
6 lettuce leaves

12 slices tomato
$^3/_4$ cup hot salsa
nonstick cooking spray

Prepare *Spicy Corn Relish* (see recipe below); cover and chill until ready to serve. Combine ground round and chili powder and mix well. Shape mixture into 6 patties. Coat grill rack with cooking spray; place on grill over medium-hot coals. Place meat patties on rack. Grill, covered, 4 minutes on each side or until done. Grill bun halves, cut sides down, 1 minute or just until toasted. To serve, line bottom half of each bun with 1 lettuce leaf; top with 2 tomato slices and a meat patty. Top each patty with 2 tablespoons salsa and 2 tablespoons *Spicy Corn Relish*. Reserve remaining corn relish for other uses. Top with remaining bun halves. Serve with roasted potato wedges. Serves 6.

Spicy Corn Relish

(1) 11-oz. can Mexican-style corn
3 tbsp. hot salsa

2 tbsp. fresh lime juice
1 tsp. ground cumin

Drain corn. Combine all ingredients; cover and chill until ready to serve.

Nutritional Information: 509 calories; 18g fat (30.4% calories from fat); 25g protein; 66g carbohydrate; 7g dietary fiber; 52mg cholesterol; 655mg sodium.

DAY 7

Breakfast

1 cup Cheerios® cereal (or high-
fiber cereal of your choice)

1 cup skim milk
2 tbsp. raisins

Nutritional Information: 249 calories; 2g fat (7.8% calories from fat); 12g protein; 49g carbohydrate; 3g dietary fiber; 4mg cholesterol; 412mg sodium.

Lunch

Tortilla Soup

(3) 6-inch fat-free flour tortillas,
cut in $^1/_2$-inch strips

2 cups chicken broth
$^1/_4$ tsp. salt

(1) 4-oz. can whole tomatoes
1/2 small onion, chopped
1/2 clove garlic, chopped
nonstick cooking spray

1 tbsp. cilantro
2 tbsp. Monterrey Jack cheese, shredded

Fry tortilla strips in heated skilled well coated with nonstick cooking spray. Puree tomatoes, onions and garlic. Bring chicken broth to a boil in a two-quart saucepan. Stir in tomato puree, salt and cilantro. Reduce heat and simmer for 10 minutes. Add half of the tortilla strips to soup. Garnish with cheese and remaining tortilla strips to serve. Serves 1.

Nutritional Information: 345 calories; 7g fat (17% calories from fat); 14g protein; 59g carbohydrate; 5g dietary fiber; 0mg cholesterol; 1,798mg sodium.

Dinner

Chicken Curry

1 lb. boneless, skinless chicken
   breasts cut into strips
1 tbsp. canola oil
1 tbsp. chopped garlic
1 medium onion, chopped
2 cups Granny Smith apples, diced

1/2 cup raisins
1 1/2 cup chicken broth, divided
2 tbsp. flour
1/8 tsp. black pepper
1/4 tsp. salt (optional)
1 tbsp. curry

In medium skillet, heat oil over medium heat and stir-fry chicken with onion and garlic until chicken is browned. Add curry, apple, raisins, salt (optional) and 1 cup of the broth. Cover and simmer for 10 minutes or until chicken is done. In a covered container, shake flour with remaining broth, or whisk together until there are no lumps. Stir into chicken mixture and bring to a boil, stirring constantly until thickened. Serve each piece over 1/2 cup cooked brown rice, 1 cup cooked green beans and wheat toast points made from sliced whole-wheat bread. Serves 4.

Nutritional Information: 579 calories; 11g fat (16.4% calories from fat); 40g protein; 84g carbohydrate; 12g dietary fiber; 66mg cholesterol; 912mg sodium.

Second Week Grocery List

Produce
- ❑ apples
- ❑ bananas
- ❑ broccoli
- ❑ cherry tomatoes
- ❑ celery
- ❑ cucumbers
- ❑ green bell pepper
- ❑ green grapes
- ❑ green onions
- ❑ green tomatoes
- ❑ Italian green beans
- ❑ lettuce
- ❑ onions
- ❑ orange
- ❑ pears
- ❑ pineapple
- ❑ plums
- ❑ potatoes
- ❑ red bell pepper
- ❑ spinach
- ❑ strawberries
- ❑ tomatoes
- ❑ zucchini
- ❑ cinnamon
- ❑ cornmeal, self-rising
- ❑ cumin, ground
- ❑ Dijon mustard
- ❑ flour
- ❑ garlic
- ❑ lime juice
- ❑ nonstick cooking spray
- ❑ nutmeg
- ❑ orange marmalade, reduced-sugar
- ❑ paprika
- ❑ raisins
- ❑ ranch dressing, light
- ❑ sage, dried
- ❑ salsa
- ❑ salt
- ❑ stuffing mix, seasoned (1 pkg.)
- ❑ Tabasco sauce
- ❑ thyme, dried
- ❑ vinaigrette dressing, light
- ❑ walnuts
- ❑ wheat germ
- ❑ Worcestershire sauce

Baking Products
- ❑ all-fruit apricot jam
- ❑ all-fruit spread (strawberry)
- ❑ balsamic vinegar
- ❑ basil
- ❑ bay leaves
- ❑ black pepper
- ❑ bouillon granules, beef-flavored
- ❑ canola oil
- ❑ cayenne pepper
- ❑ chili powder

Breads and Cereals
- ❑ bagels, whole-wheat
- ❑ bread, white
- ❑ bread, whole-wheat
- ❑ cornbread
- ❑ dinner rolls
- ❑ flour tortillas, reduced-fat
- ❑ French bread
- ❑ Grape Nuts® cereal
- ❑ oatmeal
- ❑ pasta

- ❑ pita pockets, whole-wheat
- ❑ rice
- ❑ rotini pasta

Canned Foods
- ❑ chicken broth
- ❑ Mandarin oranges (2 cans)
- ❑ marinara sauce
- ❑ mushroom soup, reduced-fat (1 can)
- ❑ peaches, in juice
- ❑ stewed tomatoes (2 cans)

Dairy Products
- ❑ blue cheese
- ❑ cheddar cheese, 2-percent
- ❑ cottage cheese, 2-percent
- ❑ cream cheese, reduced-fat
- ❑ eggs
- ❑ egg substitute
- ❑ feta cheese
- ❑ margarine, light
- ❑ mayonnaise, light
- ❑ milk, fat-free
- ❑ Mozzarella cheese, reduced-fat
- ❑ orange juice
- ❑ sour cream, light

- ❑ yogurt, plain or vanilla nonfat with sugar substitute

Frozen Foods
- ❑ okra (1 pkg.)
- ❑ pancakes, lowfat
- ❑ Stouffer's Lean Cuisine Comfort Classic® meal

Meat and Poultry
- ❑ chicken or turkey (4 oz.)
- ❑ chicken breasts (8 oz.)
- ❑ (4) chicken breasts, boneless (4 oz. each)
- ❑ (4) chicken breasts, boneless and skinless (4 oz. each)
- ❑ 1 lb. chicken breasts, boneless and skinless
- ❑ 1 lb. mixed seafood (scallops, crab, firm fish, deveined shrimp)
- ❑ (4) pork loin chops, boneless (4 oz. each)
- ❑ roasted chicken
- ❑ $3/_4$ lb. top-round steak, lean and boneless
- ❑ turkey bacon

Second Week Meals and Recipes

DAY 1

Breakfast

2 slices whole-wheat toast
2 tsp. all-fruit spread
1 cup nonfat plain or vanilla
  yogurt with sugar substitute

3 tbsp. wheat germ or 2 tbsp.
  Grape Nuts® cereal
6 oz. calcium-fortified
  orange juice

Nutritional Information: 434 calories; 5g fat (10.2% calories from fat); 22g protein; 80g carbohydrate; 8g dietary fiber; 3mg cholesterol; 433mg sodium.

Lunch

Pasta Salad
6 oz. uncooked rotini pasta
4 oz. feta cheese or blue cheese
4 oz. chicken or turkey, cooked
  and diced

1 cup celery, sliced
1 cup red bell pepper, sliced
$1/4$ cup onion, chopped
1 cup cherry tomatoes, halved

Dressing:
$1/3$ cup light mayonnaise
1 tbsp. Dijon mustard
$1/4$ cup balsamic vinegar

$1/4$ tsp. black pepper
$1/8$ tsp. basil

Cook pasta according to directions. Drain and cool. Mix all dressing ingredients until smooth. Mix pasta with remaining ingredients and garnish with cherry tomatoes. Chill before serving. Serves 4.

Nutritional Information: 383 calories; 14g fat (33% calories from fat); 20g protein; 45g carbohydrate; 3g dietary fiber; 60mg cholesterol; 568mg sodium.

Dinner

Chicken Fajitas
1 lb. boneless, skinless chicken breasts
2 tsp. canola oil
3 tbsp. lime juice
$1/2$ tsp. ground cumin
2 cups chunky salsa

1 green bell pepper, sliced
1 medium onion, sliced
(8) 6-inch reduced-fat flour tortillas
$1/2$ cup light sour cream
$1/2$ tsp. chili powder

Cut chicken breasts into 1-inch strips. Mix canola oil, lime juice, cumin and chili powder and pour over chicken. Set aside. Add vegetables to chicken and mix well. Stir-fry mixture in a skillet until done. In a separate skillet, heat tortillas and fill each with chicken mixture. Serve with salsa and sour cream. Makes 4 servings (2 filled tortillas each).

Nutritional Information: 495 calories; 10g fat (17.4% calories from fat); 37g protein; 67g carbohydrate; 7g dietary fiber; 68mg cholesterol; 1,408mg sodium.

DAY 2

Breakfast

Breakfast Burrito

$1/_2$ cup egg substitute
2 tbsp. onion, chopped
2 tbsp. bell pepper, chopped

2 tbsp. salsa
(2) 6-inch reduced-fat flour tortillas
nonstick cooking spray

Spray pan with nonstick cooking spray. Add egg substitute and scramble, then add onion and bell pepper. Place into tortillas and pour on salsa. Serve with 1 small orange. Serves 1.

Nutritional Information: 555 calories; 19g fat (29.6% calories from fat); 24g protein; 76g carbohydrate; 8g dietary fiber; 2mg cholesterol; 1,141mg sodium.

Lunch

McDonald's Premier Caesar Salad® with grilled chicken
1 pkg. lowfat dressing

1 small lowfat frozen yogurt cup
1 cup carrot sticks
1 small pear or apple

Nutritional Information: 532 calories; 10g fat (16.2% calories from fat); 38g protein; 78g carbohydrate; 11g dietary fiber; 87mg cholesterol; 1,019mg sodium.

Dinner

Stuffed Chicken Breasts

(4) 4-oz. boneless chicken breasts
$1/_2$ cup onion, chopped
$1/_2$ cup celery, chopped

$1/_8$ tsp. black pepper
1 can reduced-fat mushroom
  soup

1¹/₂ cup chicken broth
4 cups seasoned stuffing mix

¹/₂ cup water
nonstick cooking spray

Preheat oven to 350°F. In a large saucepan, combine onion, celery and broth. Simmer until vegetables are soft. Add stuffing mix and pepper. Mix well and set aside. Place each breast between plastic wrap and pound breast to about ¹/₄-inch thick. Divide stuffing mixture between each breast. Wrap breast around stuffing. Place stuffed breasts in a 9" x 9" pan that has been sprayed with nonstick cooking spray. Add ¹/₂ cup water to soup and pour over chicken. Bake covered for about 30 minutes or until chicken is no longer pink. Serve each with 1 cup broccoli. Serves 4.

Nutritional Information: 673 calories; 8g fat (11% calories from fat); 47g protein; 102g carbohydrate; 7g dietary fiber; 78mg cholesterol; 3,583mg sodium.

DAY 3

Breakfast

(1) 2-oz. whole-wheat bagel
1 tbsp. reduced-fat cream cheese

3 plums
1 cup fat-free milk

Nutritional Information: 372 calories; 5g fat (11.1% calories from fat); 17g protein; 69g carbohydrate; 5g dietary fiber; 12mg cholesterol; 493mg sodium.

Lunch

Fruited Chicken Salad

8 oz. chicken breasts, cooked
  and diced
¹/₄ cup celery, diced
mixed lettuce leaves
4 tomatoes, quartered

1 small apple, diced
¹/₂ cup grapes, halved
¹/₂ cup Mandarin orange slices
2 walnut halves, chopped
¹/₃ cup light mayonnaise

Combine cooked chicken breasts, celery, apple, grapes, Mandarin orange slices, walnuts and mayonnaise. Chill and serve on lettuce with tomatoes. Serve with 8 wheat crackers per serving. Serves 4.

Nutritional Information: 318 calories; 12g fat (33% calories from fat); 18g protein; 37g carbohydrate; 4g dietary fiber; 46mg cholesterol; 463mg sodium.

Dinner

Yogurt Cumin Chicken

(4) 4-oz. boneless, skinless
  chicken breasts
1 cup green grapes
nonstick cooking spray

3 tbsp. all-fruit apricot jam
1 tsp. ground cumin
8 oz. plain nonfat yogurt

Preheat oven to 350°F. Arrange chicken in a 9″ x 9″ pan coated with nonstick cooking spray. Bake uncovered for 20 minutes. Mix yogurt, jam and cumin and spoon over chicken. Bake for an additional 10 minutes. Garnish with grapes prior to serving. Serve each with baked zucchini and 3/4 cup of cooked pasta with 1/2 cup marinara sauce and 1 dinner roll. Serves 4.

Nutritional Information: 577 calories; 10g fat (15.2% calories from fat); 42g protein; 79g carbohydrate; 8g dietary fiber; 67mg cholesterol; 1,302mg sodium.

DAY 4

Breakfast

1 cup cooked oatmeal with a dash
  of cinnamon and nutmeg

2 tbsp. raisins
1 cup fat-free milk

Nutritional Information: 278 calories; 3g fat (9% calories from fat); 15g protein; 50g carbohydrate; 5g dietary fiber; 4mg cholesterol; 505mg sodium.

Lunch

Veggie Pita Sandwich

(1) 7-inch whole-wheat pita pocket
8 cucumber slices
4 tomato slices
1/2 tbsp. light ranch dressing

1 oz. 2-percent cheddar
  cheese, sliced

Cut pita in half. Divide all ingredients in half and fill each half of the pita. Serve with 1 small apple.

Nutritional Information: 252 calories; 4g fat (14.2% calories from fat); 15g protein; 42g carbohydrate; 7g dietary fiber; 6mg cholesterol; 533mg sodium.

Dinner

Roasted chicken

1/2 cup mashed potatoes

1 cup Italian green beans

1 dinner roll

1 tsp. light margarine

Pick up your favorite roasted chicken from the store and remove the skin before eating. Serve with potatoes, green beans and dinner roll with light margarine. Serves 4.

Nutritional Information: 595 calories; 39g fat (58.9% calories from fat); 32g protein; 28g carbohydrate; 3g dietary fiber; 115mg cholesterol; 552mg sodium.

DAY 5

Breakfast

(3) 4-inch lowfat pancakes

1 tsp. strawberry all-fruit
  spread, melted

6 oz. nonfat plain yogurt

1/2 cup fresh strawberries, chopped

Combine all-fruit spread with yogurt and strawberries to make a pancake topping. Serves 1.

Nutritional Information: 352 calories; 3g fat (8.8% calories from fat); 16g protein; 63g carbohydrate; 3g dietary fiber; 17mg cholesterol; 848mg sodium.

Lunch

Lean Cuisine Comfort
  Classic® meal of your choice

1 banana

Nutritional Information: 349 calories; 7g fat (15.9% calories from fat); 12g protein; 66g carbohydrate; 6g dietary fiber; 40mg cholesterol; 601mg sodium.

Dinner

Seafood Gumbo

1 lb. mixed seafood (scallops, crab,
  firm fish, deveined shrimp)

1 tsp. garlic, chopped

1/2 cup onion, copped

dash of cayenne pepper

Tabasco sauce (to taste)

1 tsp. paprika

2 cup chicken broth, heated

$^1/_2$ cup celery, chopped
$^1/_2$ cup bell pepper, chopped
(1) 8-oz. pkg. frozen okra
(1) 28-oz. can stewed tomatoes,
 not drained

1 tbsp. Worcestershire sauce
1 tbsp. canola oil
4 tbsp. flour
$^1/_2$ cup water

In a medium-sized saucepan, sauté onion, celery and bell pepper over medium heat until tender. Add garlic and paprika and sauté 1 minute more. Add 1 teaspoon of flour and sauté 2 minutes; do not let burn. Add the heated broth along with the Worcestershire sauce. Bring to a boil, reduce heat and add tomatoes and okra. Let simmer over medium heat until vegetables are tender. Add seasonings. Combine flour with water in a covered container and shake well. Add to gumbo mixture and cook until bubbly. Mixture will thicken. Add seafood and continue to cook until seafood is done. Serve over $^1/_2$ cup cooked rice with 1 slice toasted French bread each. Serves 4.

Nutritional Information: 689 calories; 8g fat (10.7% calories from fat); 37g protein; 116g carbohydrate; 6g dietary fiber; 94mg cholesterol; 834mg sodium.

DAY 6

Breakfast

(1) 6-inch or 7-inch whole-wheat
 pocket pita, heated
$^1/_4$ cup 2-percent cottage cheese

$^1/_2$ cup canned peaches in
 their own juice, diced
2 tsp. walnuts, chopped

Combine cottage cheese, peaches and walnuts. Split pita in half and fill each half with $^1/_2$ of the cottage cheese mixture.

Nutritional Information: 337 calories; 6g fat (15.6% calories from fat); 17g protein; 58g carbohydrate; 7g dietary fiber; 5mg cholesterol; 477mg sodium.

Lunch

Taco Bell Beef Burrito® with
 light sour cream and salsa
1 cup carrot sticks

green salad
$^1/_2$ cup fresh pineapple, cubed

Nutritional Information: 533 calories; 20g fat (32.3% calories from fat); 19g protein; 74g carbohydrate; 15g dietary fiber; 35mg cholesterol; 1,276mg sodium.

Dinner

Hearty Beef Stew

$^3/_4$ lb. lean boneless top-round steak
$2^1/_2$ tbsp. flour
$^1/_8$ tsp. salt
$^1/_8$ tsp. black pepper
$^3/_4$ lb. new potatoes
3 stalks celery, cut diagonally
   into 1-inch pieces
2 bay leaves
$^1/_4$ cup dried thyme

2 large carrots, scraped and cut
   diagonally into 1-inch pieces
$^3/_4$ cup onion, coarsely chopped
2 tsp. beef-flavored bouillon
   granules
(1) 28-oz. can stewed tomatoes
2 cups water
$^1/_2$ tsp. dried sage
nonstick cooking spray

Trim any visible fat from steak and cut into 1-inch pieces. Combine flour, salt and pepper; dredge steak in flour mixture and set aside. Coat a sheet pan with nonstick cooking spray. Place meat on pan and coat with spray. Place in a 450°F oven and cook until meat is browned all over. In a large saucepan, mix water with remaining ingredients, stirring well. Add meat, bring to a boil, and then cover and reduce heat. Simmer for 45 minutes, stirring occasionally. (If mixture is not thick enough, thicken with a little cornstarch.) Remove bay leaves before serving. Serve with a 2" x 2" square of cornbread or 1 dinner roll and a spinach salad with tomatoes and light vinaigrette dressing. Serves 4.

Nutritional Information: 582 calories; 21g fat (32% calories from fat); 28g protein; 72g carbohydrate; 7g dietary fiber; 79mg cholesterol; 928mg sodium.

DAY 7

Breakfast

Brunch Casserole

4 slices whole-wheat bread,
   crusts removed
2 oz. turkey sausage
$^1/_4$ cup mushrooms, chopped
1 tsp. onion, chopped
3 eggs, beaten

1 cup skim milk
$^1/_4$ tsp. salt
$^1/_8$ tsp. black pepper
$^1/_8$ tsp. granulated garlic
2 oz. reduced-fat cheddar
   cheese, shredded

Line the bottom of a 9" x 9" casserole dish with the bread. Sauté sausage in a nonstick skillet until done. Remove sausage and sauté mushrooms and onions until tender. Crumble the sausage and combine with the mush-rooms and onion. Sprinkle on top of bread. Combine the eggs, milk and seasonings and pour over the bread. Sprinkle with the cheese. Cover and refrigerate overnight. In the morning, set out for 15 minutes and then bake at 350°F for 40 to 45 minutes. Cut into four equal portions and serve with $^1/_2$ grapefruit. Serves 4.

Nutritional Information: 300 calories; 12g fat (36% calories from fat); 22g protein; 27g carbohydrate; 3g dietary fiber; 183mg cholesterol; 703mg sodium.

....

Lunch

Fried Green Tomato BLT

1 medium green tomato, cut into
  $^1/_4$-inch slices
$^1/_8$ tsp. hot sauce (optional)
1 egg white, lightly beaten
$1^1/_2$ tbsp. self-rising cornmeal
2 leaves green leaf lettuce
nonstick cooking spray

(2) 1-oz. slices reduced-fat
  Mozzarella cheese
2 slices turkey bacon, cooked,
  drained, and halved
(4) 1-oz. slices white sandwich
  bread, toasted

Sprinkle tomato slices with hot sauce (if desired). Dip in egg white and dredge in cornmeal. Place slices in a single layer on a baking sheet coated with nonstick cooking spray. Lightly coat slices with nonstick cooking spray. Broil 3 inches from the heat (with electric oven door partially opened) for 3 minutes on each side or until tender and golden. Layer lettuce, cheese, turkey bacon and tomato slices on 2 slices of toast. Top with remaining 2 slices of toast. Serve immediately. Serves 2.

Nutritional Information: 302 calories; 10g fat (29% calories from fat); 17g protein; 36g carbohydrate; 3g dietary fiber; 28mg cholesterol; 651mg sodium.

....

Dinner

Orange Pork Chops

(4) 4-oz. boneless pork loin chops
1 bunch green onions, trimmed
2 tbsp. Dijon mustard
nonstick cooking spray

1/3 cup reduced-sugar
  orange marmalade
1 small can Mandarin oranges

In a small saucepan, mix marmalade and mustard. Stir over medium heat until marmalade is melted. Set aside. Drain oranges and set aside. Place chops on a broiler pan or use an outdoor grill. Broil about 4 inches from the heat for about 6 minutes. Turn chops and broil 2 more minutes. Spoon half the glaze over chops. Broil 3 to 4 minutes more or until the chops are no longer pink. Slice onions diagonally into 1-inch pieces. Spray a skillet with nonstick cooking spray and stir-fry onions 2 minutes until crisp tender. Stir in remaining glaze until heated and add oranges. Serve over chops. Serve each with $^3/_4$ cup potato salad and 1 cup grilled assorted vegetables. Serves 4.

Nutritional Information: 496 calories; 21g fat (39.7% calories from fat); 26g protein; 45g carbohydrate; 3g dietary fiber; 179mg cholesterol; 1,136mg sodium.

DESSERT RECIPES

(**Note:** You will need to add the ingredients for each of these items to the grocery lists.)

Peanut Butter Banana Pudding

1 pkg. fat-free, sugar-free French vanilla instant pudding mix
2 cups fat-free milk
$^1/_3$ cup creamy peanut butter
(1) 8-oz. carton nonfat sour cream
42 reduced-fat vanilla wafers, divided
6 small bananas, divided
(1) 8-oz. carton frozen nonfat whipped topping, thawed

Prepare pudding mix according to package directions, using a whisk and 2 cups fat-free milk. Add peanut butter and sour cream, stirring well with a wire whisk. Set aside. Line bottom of a $2^1/_2$-quart casserole dish with 14 vanilla wafers. Peel and slice 4 bananas. Top wafers with one-third each of pudding mixture, banana slices, and whipped topping. Repeat layers twice using remaining wafers, pudding mixture, banana slices and whipped topping. Cover and chill at least 2 hours. To garnish, peel and slice remaining 2 bananas; arrange slices around outer edges of dish. Serves 12.

Nutritional Information: 199 calories; 6g fat (28.8% calories from fat); 5g protein; 31g carbohydrate; 2g dietary fiber; 3mg cholesterol; 237mg sodium.

Pineapple Sherbet Fluff

(8) $^1/_2$-inch slices angel food cake, torn into pieces
4 cups pineapple sherbet
$^1/_2$ cup lemon curd
$^1/_2$ cup fresh blueberries, blackberries or raspberries

Place angel food cake pieces evenly into 8 individual dessert dishes. Scoop $1/2$ cup sherbet over cake in each dish. Top each serving with 1 tablespoon lemon curd and 1 tablespoon berries. Serve immediately. Serves 8.

Nutritional Information: 197 calories; trace fat (1.2% calories from fat); 5g protein; 45g carbohydrate; trace dietary fiber; 0mg cholesterol; 380mg sodium.

Baked Pears with Gingersnaps

(2) 16-oz. cans pear halves in
 juice, drained
$1/2$ cup apricot preserves
$1/3$ cup unsweetened orange juice
1 tbsp. lemon juice
2 tsp. sugar

$1/2$ cup coarsely chopped gingersnap
 cookies (about 8 cookies)
1 tbsp. light margarine, cut in pieces
$2^1/2$ cups vanilla lowfat
 frozen yogurt
1 tbsp. brown sugar

Arrange pear halves, cut sides down, in an 11″ x 7″ x $1^1/2$″ baking dish. Combine preserves, orange juice, lemon juice and sugar in a small bowl and pour over the pear halves. Combine gingersnaps, brown sugar and margarine and sprinkle over the pear mixture. Bake at 375°F for 35 minutes or until lightly browned. To serve, spoon pear mixture into individual dessert dishes. Top each serving with $1/4$ cup frozen yogurt. Serves 10.

Nutritional Information: 206 calories; 4g fat (16% calories from fat); 3g protein; 43g carbohydrate; 2g dietary fiber; 1mg cholesterol; 133mg sodium.

Turtle Cupcakes

(1) $20^1/2$-oz. pkg. lowfat fudge
 brownie mix
$1/4$ cup finely chopped pecans

$1/3$ cup fat-free caramel-flavored
 ice cream topping
nonstick cooking spray

Prepare brownie mix according to package directions and stir in pecans. Place paper baking cups in muffin pans and coat with nonstick cooking spray. Spoon half of batter into cups, filling each about $1/3$ full. Spoon 1 teaspoon caramel topping into center of each cupcake. In each cup, drop 1 teaspoon batter from tip of spoon, guiding the batter around the caramel topping. Top evenly with remaining batter. Bake at 350°F for 25 minutes. Remove from pans and let cool completely on wire racks. Serves 16.

Nutritional Information: 213 calories; 8g fat (35% calories from fat); 1g protein; 33g carbohydrate; trace dietary fiber; 29mg cholesterol; 150mg sodium.

SNACK RECIPES

(**Note:** You will need to add the ingredients for each of these items to the grocery lists.)

Fresh Berries with Sour Cream Sauce

2 cups sliced fresh strawberries
2 cups fresh blueberries
(1) 8-oz. carton nonfat sour cream

2 tbsp. brown sugar
$1/8$ tsp. ground cinnamon

Combine strawberries and blueberries and then spoon half of the fruit mixture into 8 individual dessert bowls. Combine sour cream, brown sugar and cinnamon and stir well. Spoon sour cream mixture evenly over fruit. Garnish with mint sprigs, if desired. Serves 8.

Nutritional Information: 58 calories; trace fat (4.1% calories from fat); 2g protein; 13g carbohydrate; 2g dietary fiber; 3mg cholesterol; 22mg sodium.

Cheesy Pizza Bites

3 cups all-purpose flour
1 tsp. sugar
1 packet rapid-rise yeast
1 cup warm water
1 tbsp. extra-virgin olive oil
3 tbsp. freshly grated Parmesan cheese
nonstick cooking spray

1 pint cherry tomatoes
4 oz. fontina cheese, shredded
12 kalamata olives, pitted and cut
   into slivers
fresh oregano leaves
$1/2$ tsp. salt

Mix 1 cup flour, sugar and yeast in a bowl. Stir in the water and oil until blended. Place $1^3/4$ cups flour and salt in a food processor and mix. Add yeast mixture and continue to mix until blended. Add remaining flour 1 tablespoon at a time until a soft dough forms (about 2 minutes). The dough will be ready when it comes together in a ball. Dust work surface lightly with flour. Turn out dough and knead until smooth (1 to 2 minutes). Roll the dough into $1^1/2$-inch balls in your hands, then flatten into 3-inch rounds. Cover with clean kitchen towel and let rest 10 minutes. Preheat oven to 450°F. Line two baking sheets with parchment paper and divide dough into 4 pieces. Wrap 3 pieces in plastic and refrigerate. Cut remaining dough into 12 equal pieces and shape each into $1^1/2$-inch ball. Arrange on baking sheets, flatten into 3-inch rounds, and lightly coat with nonstick cooking spray. Cut tomatoes into thin slices, and then fan out slices. Top each pizza with 2 or 3 slices. Sprinkle with 1 teaspoon fontina, a little Parmesan, and a few olive slivers and oregano leaves. Bake until bubbly and crust is golden (about 10 minutes). Repeat with remaining dough. Serves 12 (2 pizza bites per person).

Nutritional Information: 87 calories; 3g fat (30.1% calories from fat); 3g protein; 12g carbohydrate; 1g dietary fiber; 6mg cholesterol; 125mg sodium.

Spicy Edamame

$3/4$ cup preshelled edamame
$1/2$ tsp. sea salt

$1/4$ tsp. chili powder
(or garlic salt)

Boil edamame in small saucepan for 5 minutes. Drain. Sprinkle with sea salt and chili powder.

Nutritional Information: 180 calories; 4g fat (19% calories from fat); 17g protein; 20g carbohydrate; 14g dietary fiber; 0mg cholesterol; 23mg sodium.

Chocolate Yogurt Pops

$1^{1}/_{2}$ cups lowfat yogurt
$1/3$ cup cold water

2 pkgs. hot chocolate mix
2 tbsp. cocoa

Combine all ingredients in blender and blend. Pour into four 4-ounce ice pop molds. Freeze overnight. Serves 4.

Nutritional Information: 112 calories; 2g fat (11.3% calories from fat); 5g protein; 22g carbohydrate; 1g dietary fiber; 4mg cholesterol; 79mg sodium.

Potato Skins

2 medium russet potatoes
1 tbsp. minced fresh rosemary

$1/8$ tsp. freshly ground black pepper
nonstick cooking spray

Preheat oven to 375°F. Wash the potatoes and pierce with a fork. Place in the oven until the skins are crisp (about 1 hour). Carefully cut the potatoes in half and scoop out the pulp, leaving about $1/8$ inch of the potato flesh attached to the skin. Spray the inside of each potato skin with nonstick cooking spray. Press in the rosemary and pepper and return the skins to the oven for 5 to 10 minutes. Serve immediately. Serves 2.

Nutritional Information: 60 calories; trace fat (1.7% calories from fat); 2g protein; 14g carbohydrate; 1g dietary fiber; 0mg cholesterol; 5mg sodium.

HEALTHY SNACK OPTIONS

(**Note:** You will need to add the ingredients for each of these items to the grocery lists.)

- Apple slices with 1 tablespoon peanut butter: 200 calories.
- Banana sliced in half and spread lightly with 1 tablespoon peanut butter: 200 calories.
- Vegetables with 2 tablespoons light ranch dressing: 50 calories.
- 4 cups light popcorn sprinkled with 2 tablespoons Parmesan cheese): 120 calories.
- 1 cup red grapes with string cheese: 110 calories.
- 4 rice cakes spread very lightly with 1 tablespoon peanut butter: 235 calories.
- Small (2-oz.) bagel spread with 1 tablespoon lowfat cream cheese: 220 calories.
- String cheese with 4 whole-grain crackers: 125 calories.
- $1/4$ cup trail mix: 150 calories.
- 1 cup of vegetable soup with 4 whole-grain crackers: 125 calories.
- 1 cup whole-grain cereal with 1 cup lowfat milk: 195 calories.
- Whole-grain English muffin spread lightly with 1 tablespoon peanut butter: 230 calories.

Member Survey

Please answer the following questions to help your leader plan your First Place 4 Health meetings so that your needs might be met in this session. Give this form to your leader at the first group meeting.

Name **Emily Long**   Birth date **7/18/1976**

Please list those who live in your household.

Name	Relationship	Age
Gavin	husband	34
Jenny	sister	31
four daughters		8, 6, 3, 1

What church do you attend? **RBC**

Are you interested in receiving more information about our church?

Yes   (No)

Occupation **stay at home mom**

What talent or area of expertise would you be willing to share with our class?

singing, worship, leadership

Why did you join First Place 4 Health?

loose weight

With notice, would you be willing to lead a Bible study discussion one week?

(Yes)   No

Are you comfortable praying out loud? **yes**

If the assistant leader were absent, would you be willing to assist in weighing in members and possibly evaluating the Live It Trackers?

(Yes)   No

Any other comments:

Personal Weight and Measurement Record

Week	Weight	+ or -	Goal this Session	Pounds to goal
1	247			
2				
3				
4				
5				
6				
7				
8				
9				
10				
11				
12				

Beginning Measurements

Waist _____ Hips _____ Thighs _____ Chest _____

Ending Measurements

Waist _____ Hips _____ Thighs _____ Chest _____

First Place 4 Health
Prayer Partner

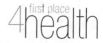

GIVING CHRIST
CONTROL
Week
1

SCRIPTURE VERSE TO MEMORIZE FOR WEEK TWO:

*Restore to me the joy of your salvation
and grant me a willing spirit, to sustain me.*

PSALM 51:12

Date: _____

Name: _____

Home Phone: (_____) _____

Work Phone: (_____) _____

Email: _____

Personal Prayer Concerns:

_____

_____

_____

_____

_____

_____

_____

This form is for prayer requests that are personal to you and your journey in First Place 4 Health. Please complete this form and have it ready to turn in when you arrive at your group meeting.

First Place 4 Health
Prayer Partner

GIVING CHRIST
CONTROL
Week
2

SCRIPTURE VERSE TO MEMORIZE FOR WEEK THREE:

*May the God of hope fill you with all joy and peace as you trust in him,
so that you may overflow with hope by the power of the Holy Spirit.*

ROMANS 15:13

Date: _____

Name: _____

Home Phone: ( ) _____

Work Phone: ( ) _____

Email: _____

Personal Prayer Concerns:

_____

_____

_____

_____

_____

_____

_____

This form is for prayer requests that are personal to you and your journey in First Place 4 Health. Please complete this form and have it ready to turn in when you arrive at your group meeting.

First Place 4 Health
Prayer Partner

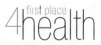

GIVING CHRIST
CONTROL
Week
3

SCRIPTURE VERSE TO MEMORIZE FOR WEEK FOUR:

*Finally, brothers, whatever is true, whatever is noble, whatever is right,
whatever is pure, whatever is lovely, whatever is admirable—if anything
is excellent or praiseworthy—think about such things.*

PHILIPPIANS 4:8

Date: _____

Name: _____

Home Phone: (_____) _____

Work Phone: (_____) _____

Email: _____

Personal Prayer Concerns:

_____

_____

_____

_____

_____

_____

_____

This form is for prayer requests that are personal to you and your journey in First Place 4 Health. Please complete this form and have it ready to turn in when you arrive at your group meeting.

First Place 4 Health
Prayer Partner

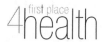

Scripture Verse to Memorize for Week Five:

*I have been crucified with Christ and I no longer live, but Christ
lives in me. The life I live in the body, I live by faith in the Son of God,
who loved me and gave himself for me.*

Galatians 2:20

Date: _____

Name: _____

Home Phone: (_____) _____

Work Phone: (_____) _____

Email: _____

Personal Prayer Concerns:

_____

_____

_____

_____

_____

_____

This form is for prayer requests that are personal to you and your journey in First Place 4 Health. Please complete this form and have it ready to turn in when you arrive at your group meeting.

First Place 4 Health
Prayer Partner

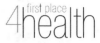

GIVING CHRIST
CONTROL
Week
5

SCRIPTURE VERSE TO MEMORIZE FOR WEEK SIX:

*I have learned the secret of being content in any and every
situation, whether well fed or hungry, whether living in plenty or in want.
I can do everything through him who gives me strength.*

PHILIPPIANS 4:12-13

Date: _____

Name: _____

Home Phone: (_____) _____

Work Phone: (_____) _____

Email: _____

Personal Prayer Concerns:

_____

_____

_____

_____

_____

_____

_____

This form is for prayer requests that are personal to you and your journey in First Place 4 Health. Please complete this form and have it ready to turn in when you arrive at your group meeting.

First Place 4 Health
Prayer Partner

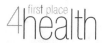

GIVING CHRIST
CONTROL
Week
6

SCRIPTURE VERSE TO MEMORIZE FOR WEEK SEVEN:

Do not think of yourself more highly than you ought,
but rather think of yourself with sober judgment,
in accordance with the measure of faith God has given you.

ROMANS 12:3

Date: _____

Name: _____

Home Phone: (_____) _____

Work Phone: (_____) _____

Email: _____

Personal Prayer Concerns:

_____

_____

_____

_____

_____

_____

_____

This form is for prayer requests that are personal to you and your journey in First Place 4 Health. Please complete this form and have it ready to turn in when you arrive at your group meeting.

First Place 4 Health
Prayer Partner

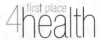

GIVING CHRIST
CONTROL
Week
7

SCRIPTURE VERSE TO MEMORIZE FOR WEEK EIGHT:

If anyone considers himself religious and yet does not keep a tight rein on his tongue, he deceives himself and his religion is worthless.

JAMES 1:26

Date: _____

Name: _____

Home Phone: (_____) _____

Work Phone: (_____) _____

Email: _____

Personal Prayer Concerns:

_____

_____

_____

_____

_____

_____

_____

This form is for prayer requests that are personal to you and your journey in First Place 4 Health. Please complete this form and have it ready to turn in when you arrive at your group meeting.

First Place 4 Health
Prayer Partner

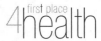

GIVING CHRIST
CONTROL
Week
8

SCRIPTURE VERSE TO MEMORIZE FOR WEEK NINE:
If anyone would come after me, he must deny
himself and take up his cross daily and follow me.

LUKE 9:23

Date: _____

Name: _____

Home Phone: (_____)_____

Work Phone: (_____)_____

Email: _____

Personal Prayer Concerns:

_____

_____

_____

_____

_____

_____

This form is for prayer requests that are personal to you and your journey in First Place 4 Health. Please complete this form and have it ready to turn in when you arrive at your group meeting.

First Place 4 Health
Prayer Partner

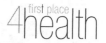

GIVING CHRIST
CONTROL
Week
9

SCRIPTURE VERSE TO MEMORIZE FOR WEEK TEN:

Let us consider how we may spur one another on toward love and good deeds.
Let us not give up meeting together, as some are in the habit of doing, but let us
encourage one another—and all the more as you see the Day approaching.

HEBREWS 10:24-25

Date: _____

Name: _____

Home Phone: (_____) _____

Work Phone: (_____) _____

Email: _____

Personal Prayer Concerns:

_____

_____

_____

_____

_____

_____

_____

This form is for prayer requests that are personal to you and your journey in First Place 4 Health. Please complete this form and have it ready to turn in when you arrive at your group meeting.

First Place 4 Health
Prayer Partner

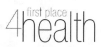

GIVING CHRIST
CONTROL
Week
10

SCRIPTURE VERSE TO MEMORIZE FOR WEEK ELEVEN:

May God himself, the God of peace, sanctify you through and through. May your whole spirit, soul and body be kept blameless at the coming of our Lord Jesus Christ.

1 THESSALONIANS 5:23

Date: _____

Name: _____

Home Phone: (_____) _____

Work Phone: (_____) _____

Email: _____

Personal Prayer Concerns:

_____

_____

_____

_____

_____

_____

This form is for prayer requests that are personal to you and your journey in First Place 4 Health. Please complete this form and have it ready to turn in when you arrive at your group meeting.

First Place 4 Health
Prayer Partner

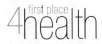

GIVING CHRIST
CONTROL
Week
11

Date: _____

Name: _____

Home Phone: (_____) _____

Work Phone: (_____) _____

Email: _____

Personal Prayer Concerns:

_____

_____

_____

_____

_____

_____

_____

This form is for prayer requests that are personal to you and your journey in First Place 4 Health. Please complete this form and have it ready to turn in when you arrive at your group meeting.

Live It Tracker

Name: Emily

Loss/gain: _____ lbs.

Date: 4/14/10 Week #: 1 Calorie Range: 2000 My food goal for next week: _____

Activity Level: None, < 30 min/day, 30-60 min/day, 60+ min/day My activity goal for next week: _____

Group	Daily Calories							
	1300-1400	1500-1600	1700-1800	1900-2000	2100-2200	2300-2400	2500-2600	2700-2800
Fruits	1.5-2 c.	1.5-2 c.	1.5-2 c.	2-2.5 c.	2-2.5 c.	2.5-3.5 c.	3.5-4.5 c.	3.5-4.5 c.
Vegetables	1.5-2 c.	2-2.5 c.	2.5-3 c.	2.5-3 c.	3-3.5 c.	3.5-4.5 c.	4.5-5 c.	4.5-5 c.
Grains	5 oz-eq.	5-6 oz-eq.	6-7 oz-eq.	6-7 oz-eq.	7-8 oz-eq.	8-9 oz-eq.	9-10 oz-eq.	10-11 oz-eq.
Meat & Beans	4 oz-eq.	5 oz-eq.	5-5.5 oz-eq.	5.5-6.5 oz-eq.	6.5-7 oz-eq.	7-7.5 oz-eq.	7-7.5 oz-eq.	7.5-8 oz-eq.
Milk	2-3 c.	3 c.	3 c.	3 c.	3 c.	3 c.	3 c.	3 c.
Healthy Oils	4 tsp.	5 tsp.	5 tsp.	6 tsp.	6 tsp.	7 tsp.	8 tsp.	8 tsp.

Day/Date: Wed, 14th

Breakfast: probiotic yogurt, granola strawberries, half small bagel, or chese Lunch: _____

Dinner: _____ Snack: _____

Group	Fruits	Vegetables	Grains	Meat & Beans	Milk	Oils
Goal Amount	1					
Estimate Your Total						
Increase ⬆ or Decrease? ⬇						

Physical Activity: _____ Spiritual Activity: _____

Steps/Miles/Minutes: _____

Day/Date:

Breakfast: _____ Lunch: _____

Dinner: _____ Snack: _____

Group	Fruits	Vegetables	Grains	Meat & Beans	Milk	Oils
Goal Amount						
Estimate Your Total						
Increase ⬆ or Decrease? ⬇						

Physical Activity: _____ Spiritual Activity: _____

Steps/Miles/Minutes: _____

Day/Date:

Breakfast: _____ Lunch: _____

Dinner: _____ Snack: _____

Group	Fruits	Vegetables	Grains	Meat & Beans	Milk	Oils
Goal Amount						
Estimate Your Total						
Increase ⬆ or Decrease? ⬇						

Physical Activity: _____ Spiritual Activity: _____

Steps/Miles/Minutes: _____

Day/Date:

Breakfast: _____   Lunch: _____
_____
Dinner: _____   Snack: _____
_____

Group	Fruits	Vegetables	Grains	Meat & Beans	Milk	Oils
Goal Amount						
Estimate Your Total						
Increase ⇧ or Decrease? ⇩						

Physical Activity: _____   Spiritual Activity: _____
Steps/Miles/Minutes: _____   _____

Day/Date:

Breakfast: _____   Lunch: _____
_____
Dinner: _____   Snack: _____
_____

Group	Fruits	Vegetables	Grains	Meat & Beans	Milk	Oils
Goal Amount						
Estimate Your Total						
Increase ⇧ or Decrease? ⇩						

Physical Activity: _____   Spiritual Activity: _____
Steps/Miles/Minutes: _____   _____

Day/Date:

Breakfast: _____   Lunch: _____
_____
Dinner: _____   Snack: _____
_____

Group	Fruits	Vegetables	Grains	Meat & Beans	Milk	Oils
Goal Amount						
Estimate Your Total						
Increase ⇧ or Decrease? ⇩						

Physical Activity: _____   Spiritual Activity: _____
Steps/Miles/Minutes: _____   _____

Day/Date:

Breakfast: _____   Lunch: _____
_____
Dinner: _____   Snack: _____
_____

Group	Fruits	Vegetables	Grains	Meat & Beans	Milk	Oils
Goal Amount						
Estimate Your Total						
Increase ⇧ or Decrease? ⇩						

Physical Activity: _____   Spiritual Activity: _____
Steps/Miles/Minutes: _____   _____

Live It Tracker

Name: _____ Loss/gain: _____ lbs.

Date: _____ Week #: _____ Calorie Range: _____ My food goal for next week: _____

Activity Level: None, < 30 min/day, 30-60 min/day, 60+ min/day   My activity goal for next week: _____

Group	Daily Calories							
	1300-1400	1500-1600	1700-1800	1900-2000	2100-2200	2300-2400	2500-2600	2700-2800
Fruits	1.5-2 c.	1.5-2 c.	1.5-2 c.	2-2.5 c.	2-2.5 c.	2.5-3.5 c.	3.5-4.5 c.	3.5-4.5 c.
Vegetables	1.5-2 c.	2-2.5 c.	2.5-3 c.	2.5-3 c.	3-3.5 c.	3.5-4.5 c.	4.5-5 c.	4.5-5 c.
Grains	5 oz-eq.	5-6 oz-eq.	6-7 oz-eq.	6-7 oz-eq.	7-8 oz-eq.	8-9 oz-eq.	9-10 oz-eq.	10-11 oz-eq.
Meat & Beans	4 oz-eq.	5 oz-eq.	5-5.5 oz-eq.	5.5-6.5 oz-eq.	6.5-7 oz-eq.	7-7.5 oz-eq.	7-7.5 oz-eq.	7.5-8 oz-eq.
Milk	2-3 c.	3 c.	3 c.	3 c.	3 c.	3 c.	3 c.	3 c.
Healthy Oils	4 tsp.	5 tsp.	5 tsp.	6 tsp.	6 tsp.	7 tsp.	8 tsp.	8 tsp.

Day/Date:

Breakfast: _____   Lunch: _____

Dinner: _____   Snack: _____

Group	Fruits	Vegetables	Grains	Meat & Beans	Milk	Oils
Goal Amount						
Estimate Your Total						
Increase ⇧ or Decrease? ⇩						

Physical Activity: _____   Spiritual Activity: _____

Steps/Miles/Minutes: _____

Day/Date:

Breakfast: _____   Lunch: _____

Dinner: _____   Snack: _____

Group	Fruits	Vegetables	Grains	Meat & Beans	Milk	Oils
Goal Amount						
Estimate Your Total						
Increase ⇧ or Decrease? ⇩						

Physical Activity: _____   Spiritual Activity: _____

Steps/Miles/Minutes: _____

Day/Date:

Breakfast: _____   Lunch: _____

Dinner: _____   Snack: _____

Group	Fruits	Vegetables	Grains	Meat & Beans	Milk	Oils
Goal Amount						
Estimate Your Total						
Increase ⇧ or Decrease? ⇩						

Physical Activity: _____   Spiritual Activity: _____

Steps/Miles/Minutes: _____

Day/Date: _____

Breakfast: _____ Lunch: _____

Dinner: _____ Snack: _____

Group	Fruits	Vegetables	Grains	Meat & Beans	Milk	Oils
Goal Amount						
Estimate Your Total						
Increase ⇧ or Decrease? ⇩						

Physical Activity: _____ Spiritual Activity: _____

Steps/Miles/Minutes: _____

Day/Date: _____

Breakfast: _____ Lunch: _____

Dinner: _____ Snack: _____

Group	Fruits	Vegetables	Grains	Meat & Beans	Milk	Oils
Goal Amount						
Estimate Your Total						
Increase ⇧ or Decrease? ⇩						

Physical Activity: _____ Spiritual Activity: _____

Steps/Miles/Minutes: _____

Day/Date: _____

Breakfast: _____ Lunch: _____

Dinner: _____ Snack: _____

Group	Fruits	Vegetables	Grains	Meat & Beans	Milk	Oils
Goal Amount						
Estimate Your Total						
Increase ⇧ or Decrease? ⇩						

Physical Activity: _____ Spiritual Activity: _____

Steps/Miles/Minutes: _____

Day/Date: _____

Breakfast: _____ Lunch: _____

Dinner: _____ Snack: _____

Group	Fruits	Vegetables	Grains	Meat & Beans	Milk	Oils
Goal Amount						
Estimate Your Total						
Increase ⇧ or Decrease? ⇩						

Physical Activity: _____ Spiritual Activity: _____

Steps/Miles/Minutes: _____

Live It Tracker

Name: _____ Loss/gain: _____ lbs.

Date: _____ Week #: _____ Calorie Range: _____ My food goal for next week: _____

Activity Level: None, < 30 min/day, 30-60 min/day, 60+ min/day   My activity goal for next week: _____

Group	Daily Calories							
	1300-1400	1500-1600	1700-1800	1900-2000	2100-2200	2300-2400	2500-2600	2700-2800
Fruits	1.5-2 c.	1.5-2 c.	1.5-2 c.	2-2.5 c.	2-2.5 c.	2.5-3.5 c.	3.5-4.5 c.	3.5-4.5 c.
Vegetables	1.5-2 c.	2-2.5 c.	2.5-3 c.	2.5-3 c.	3-3.5 c.	3.5-4.5 c.	4.5-5 c.	4.5-5 c.
Grains	5 oz-eq.	5-6 oz-eq.	6-7 oz-eq.	6-7 oz-eq.	7-8 oz-eq.	8-9 oz-eq.	9-10 oz-eq.	10-11 oz-eq.
Meat & Beans	4 oz-eq.	5 oz-eq.	5-5.5 oz-eq.	5.5-6.5 oz-eq.	6.5-7 oz-eq.	7-7.5 oz-eq.	7-7.5 oz-eq.	7.5-8 oz-eq.
Milk	2-3 c.	3 c.	3 c.	3 c.	3 c.	3 c.	3 c.	3 c.
Healthy Oils	4 tsp.	5 tsp.	5 tsp.	6 tsp.	6 tsp.	7 tsp.	8 tsp.	8 tsp.

Day/Date:

Breakfast: _____   Lunch: _____

Dinner: _____   Snack: _____

Group	Fruits	Vegetables	Grains	Meat & Beans	Milk	Oils
Goal Amount						
Estimate Your Total						
Increase ⇧ or Decrease? ⇩						

Physical Activity: _____   Spiritual Activity: _____

Steps/Miles/Minutes: _____

Day/Date:

Breakfast: _____   Lunch: _____

Dinner: _____   Snack: _____

Group	Fruits	Vegetables	Grains	Meat & Beans	Milk	Oils
Goal Amount						
Estimate Your Total						
Increase ⇧ or Decrease? ⇩						

Physical Activity: _____   Spiritual Activity: _____

Steps/Miles/Minutes: _____

Day/Date:

Breakfast: _____   Lunch: _____

Dinner: _____   Snack: _____

Group	Fruits	Vegetables	Grains	Meat & Beans	Milk	Oils
Goal Amount						
Estimate Your Total						
Increase ⇧ or Decrease? ⇩						

Physical Activity: _____   Spiritual Activity: _____

Steps/Miles/Minutes: _____

Day/Date: _____

Breakfast: _____ Lunch: _____

Dinner: _____ Snack: _____

Group	Fruits	Vegetables	Grains	Meat & Beans	Milk	Oils
Goal Amount						
Estimate Your Total						
Increase ⬆ or Decrease? ⬇						

Physical Activity: _____ Spiritual Activity: _____

Steps/Miles/Minutes: _____

Day/Date: _____

Breakfast: _____ Lunch: _____

Dinner: _____ Snack: _____

Group	Fruits	Vegetables	Grains	Meat & Beans	Milk	Oils
Goal Amount						
Estimate Your Total						
Increase ⬆ or Decrease? ⬇						

Physical Activity: _____ Spiritual Activity: _____

Steps/Miles/Minutes: _____

Day/Date: _____

Breakfast: _____ Lunch: _____

Dinner: _____ Snack: _____

Group	Fruits	Vegetables	Grains	Meat & Beans	Milk	Oils
Goal Amount						
Estimate Your Total						
Increase ⬆ or Decrease? ⬇						

Physical Activity: _____ Spiritual Activity: _____

Steps/Miles/Minutes: _____

Day/Date: _____

Breakfast: _____ Lunch: _____

Dinner: _____ Snack: _____

Group	Fruits	Vegetables	Grains	Meat & Beans	Milk	Oils
Goal Amount						
Estimate Your Total						
Increase ⬆ or Decrease? ⬇						

Physical Activity: _____ Spiritual Activity: _____

Steps/Miles/Minutes: _____

Live It Tracker

Name: _____ Loss/gain: _____ lbs.

Date: _____ Week #: ____ Calorie Range: _____ My food goal for next week: _____

Activity Level: None, < 30 min/day, 30-60 min/day, 60+ min/day My activity goal for next week: _____

Group	Daily Calories							
	1300-1400	1500-1600	1700-1800	1900-2000	2100-2200	2300-2400	2500-2600	2700-2800
Fruits	1.5-2 c.	1.5-2 c.	1.5-2 c.	2-2.5 c.	2-2.5 c.	2.5-3.5 c.	3.5-4.5 c.	3.5-4.5 c.
Vegetables	1.5-2 c.	2-2.5 c.	2.5-3 c.	2.5-3 c.	3-3.5 c.	3.5-4.5 c.	4.5-5 c.	4.5-5 c.
Grains	5 oz-eq.	5-6 oz-eq.	6-7 oz-eq.	6-7 oz-eq.	7-8 oz-eq.	8-9 oz-eq.	9-10 oz-eq.	10-11 oz-eq.
Meat & Beans	4 oz-eq.	5 oz-eq.	5-5.5 oz-eq.	5.5-6.5 oz-eq.	6.5-7 oz-eq.	7-7.5 oz-eq.	7-7.5 oz-eq.	7.5-8 oz-eq.
Milk	2-3 c.	3 c.	3 c.	3 c.	3 c.	3 c.	3 c.	3 c.
Healthy Oils	4 tsp.	5 tsp.	5 tsp.	6 tsp.	6 tsp.	7 tsp.	8 tsp.	8 tsp.

Day/Date:

Breakfast: _____ Lunch: _____

Dinner: _____ Snack: _____

Group	Fruits	Vegetables	Grains	Meat & Beans	Milk	Oils
Goal Amount						
Estimate Your Total						
Increase ⇧ or Decrease? ⇩						

Physical Activity: _____ Spiritual Activity: _____

Steps/Miles/Minutes: _____

Day/Date:

Breakfast: _____ Lunch: _____

Dinner: _____ Snack: _____

Group	Fruits	Vegetables	Grains	Meat & Beans	Milk	Oils
Goal Amount						
Estimate Your Total						
Increase ⇧ or Decrease? ⇩						

Physical Activity: _____ Spiritual Activity: _____

Steps/Miles/Minutes: _____

Day/Date:

Breakfast: _____ Lunch: _____

Dinner: _____ Snack: _____

Group	Fruits	Vegetables	Grains	Meat & Beans	Milk	Oils
Goal Amount						
Estimate Your Total						
Increase ⇧ or Decrease? ⇩						

Physical Activity: _____ Spiritual Activity: _____

Steps/Miles/Minutes: _____

Day/Date: _____

Breakfast: _____ Lunch: _____
_____
Dinner: _____ Snack: _____
_____

Group	Fruits	Vegetables	Grains	Meat & Beans	Milk	Oils
Goal Amount						
Estimate Your Total						
Increase ⇧ or Decrease? ⇩						

Physical Activity: _____ Spiritual Activity: _____
Steps/Miles/Minutes: _____ _____

Day/Date: _____

Breakfast: _____ Lunch: _____
_____
Dinner: _____ Snack: _____
_____

Group	Fruits	Vegetables	Grains	Meat & Beans	Milk	Oils
Goal Amount						
Estimate Your Total						
Increase ⇧ or Decrease? ⇩						

Physical Activity: _____ Spiritual Activity: _____
Steps/Miles/Minutes: _____ _____

Day/Date: _____

Breakfast: _____ Lunch: _____
_____
Dinner: _____ Snack: _____
_____

Group	Fruits	Vegetables	Grains	Meat & Beans	Milk	Oils
Goal Amount						
Estimate Your Total						
Increase ⇧ or Decrease? ⇩						

Physical Activity: _____ Spiritual Activity: _____
Steps/Miles/Minutes: _____ _____

Day/Date: _____

Breakfast: _____ Lunch: _____
_____
Dinner: _____ Snack: _____
_____

Group	Fruits	Vegetables	Grains	Meat & Beans	Milk	Oils
Goal Amount						
Estimate Your Total						
Increase ⇧ or Decrease? ⇩						

Physical Activity: _____ Spiritual Activity: _____
Steps/Miles/Minutes: _____ _____

Live It Tracker

Name: _____   Loss/gain: _____ lbs.

Date: _____ Week #: _____ Calorie Range: _____ My food goal for next week: _____

Activity Level: None, < 30 min/day, 30-60 min/day, 60+ min/day   My activity goal for next week: _____

Group	Daily Calories							
	1300-1400	1500-1600	1700-1800	1900-2000	2100-2200	2300-2400	2500-2600	2700-2800
Fruits	1.5-2 c.	1.5-2 c.	1.5-2 c.	2-2.5 c.	2-2.5 c.	2.5-3.5 c.	3.5-4.5 c.	3.5-4.5 c.
Vegetables	1.5-2 c.	2-2.5 c.	2.5-3 c.	2.5-3 c.	3-3.5 c.	3.5-4.5 c.	4.5-5 c.	4.5-5 c.
Grains	5 oz-eq.	5-6 oz-eq.	6-7 oz-eq.	6-7 oz-eq.	7-8 oz-eq.	8-9 oz-eq.	9-10 oz-eq.	10-11 oz-eq.
Meat & Beans	4 oz-eq.	5 oz-eq.	5-5.5 oz-eq.	5.5-6.5 oz-eq.	6.5-7 oz-eq.	7-7.5 oz-eq.	7-7.5 oz-eq.	7.5-8 oz-eq.
Milk	2-3 c.	3 c.	3 c.	3 c.	3 c.	3 c.	3 c.	3 c.
Healthy Oils	4 tsp.	5 tsp.	5 tsp.	6 tsp.	6 tsp.	7 tsp.	8 tsp.	8 tsp.

Day/Date:

Breakfast: _____   Lunch: _____

Dinner: _____   Snack: _____

Group	Fruits	Vegetables	Grains	Meat & Beans	Milk	Oils
Goal Amount						
Estimate Your Total						
Increase ⇧ or Decrease? ⇩						

Physical Activity: _____   Spiritual Activity: _____

Steps/Miles/Minutes: _____

Day/Date:

Breakfast: _____   Lunch: _____

Dinner: _____   Snack: _____

Group	Fruits	Vegetables	Grains	Meat & Beans	Milk	Oils
Goal Amount						
Estimate Your Total						
Increase ⇧ or Decrease? ⇩						

Physical Activity: _____   Spiritual Activity: _____

Steps/Miles/Minutes: _____

Day/Date:

Breakfast: _____   Lunch: _____

Dinner: _____   Snack: _____

Group	Fruits	Vegetables	Grains	Meat & Beans	Milk	Oils
Goal Amount						
Estimate Your Total						
Increase ⇧ or Decrease? ⇩						

Physical Activity: _____   Spiritual Activity: _____

Steps/Miles/Minutes: _____

Day/Date: _____

Breakfast: _____ Lunch: _____

Dinner: _____ Snack: _____

Group	Fruits	Vegetables	Grains	Meat & Beans	Milk	Oils
Goal Amount						
Estimate Your Total						
Increase ⬆ or Decrease? ⬇						

Physical Activity: _____ Spiritual Activity: _____

Steps/Miles/Minutes: _____ _____

Day/Date: _____

Breakfast: _____ Lunch: _____

Dinner: _____ Snack: _____

Group	Fruits	Vegetables	Grains	Meat & Beans	Milk	Oils
Goal Amount						
Estimate Your Total						
Increase ⬆ or Decrease? ⬇						

Physical Activity: _____ Spiritual Activity: _____

Steps/Miles/Minutes: _____ _____

Day/Date: _____

Breakfast: _____ Lunch: _____

Dinner: _____ Snack: _____

Group	Fruits	Vegetables	Grains	Meat & Beans	Milk	Oils
Goal Amount						
Estimate Your Total						
Increase ⬆ or Decrease? ⬇						

Physical Activity: _____ Spiritual Activity: _____

Steps/Miles/Minutes: _____ _____

Day/Date: _____

Breakfast: _____ Lunch: _____

Dinner: _____ Snack: _____

Group	Fruits	Vegetables	Grains	Meat & Beans	Milk	Oils
Goal Amount						
Estimate Your Total						
Increase ⬆ or Decrease? ⬇						

Physical Activity: _____ Spiritual Activity: _____

Steps/Miles/Minutes: _____ _____

Live It Tracker

Name: _____   Loss/gain: _____ lbs.

Date: _____ Week #: ____ Calorie Range: _____ My food goal for next week: _____

Activity Level: None, < 30 min/day, 30-60 min/day, 60+ min/day My activity goal for next week: _____

Group	Daily Calories							
	1300-1400	1500-1600	1700-1800	1900-2000	2100-2200	2300-2400	2500-2600	2700-2800
Fruits	1.5-2 c.	1.5-2 c.	1.5-2 c.	2-2.5 c.	2-2.5 c.	2.5-3.5 c.	3.5-4.5 c.	3.5-4.5 c.
Vegetables	1.5-2 c.	2-2.5 c.	2.5-3 c.	2.5-3 c.	3-3.5 c.	3.5-4.5 c.	4.5-5 c.	4.5-5 c.
Grains	5 oz-eq.	5-6 oz-eq.	6-7 oz-eq.	6-7 oz-eq.	7-8 oz-eq.	8-9 oz-eq.	9-10 oz-eq.	10-11 oz-eq.
Meat & Beans	4 oz-eq.	5 oz-eq.	5-5.5 oz-eq.	5.5-6.5 oz-eq.	6.5-7 oz-eq.	7-7.5 oz-eq.	7-7.5 oz-eq.	7.5-8 oz-eq.
Milk	2-3 c.	3 c.	3 c.	3 c.	3 c.	3 c.	3 c.	3 c.
Healthy Oils	4 tsp.	5 tsp.	5 tsp.	6 tsp.	6 tsp.	7 tsp.	8 tsp.	8 tsp.

Day/Date:

Breakfast: _____   Lunch: _____

Dinner: _____   Snack: _____

Group	Fruits	Vegetables	Grains	Meat & Beans	Milk	Oils
Goal Amount						
Estimate Your Total						
Increase ⇧ or Decrease? ⇩						

Physical Activity: _____   Spiritual Activity: _____

Steps/Miles/Minutes: _____

Day/Date:

Breakfast: _____   Lunch: _____

Dinner: _____   Snack: _____

Group	Fruits	Vegetables	Grains	Meat & Beans	Milk	Oils
Goal Amount						
Estimate Your Total						
Increase ⇧ or Decrease? ⇩						

Physical Activity: _____   Spiritual Activity: _____

Steps/Miles/Minutes: _____

Day/Date:

Breakfast: _____   Lunch: _____

Dinner: _____   Snack: _____

Group	Fruits	Vegetables	Grains	Meat & Beans	Milk	Oils
Goal Amount						
Estimate Your Total						
Increase ⇧ or Decrease? ⇩						

Physical Activity: _____   Spiritual Activity: _____

Steps/Miles/Minutes: _____

Day/Date: _____

Breakfast: _____ Lunch: _____

Dinner: _____ Snack: _____

Group	Fruits	Vegetables	Grains	Meat & Beans	Milk	Oils
Goal Amount						
Estimate Your Total						
Increase ⇧ or Decrease? ⇩						

Physical Activity: _____ Spiritual Activity: _____

Steps/Miles/Minutes: _____ _____

Day/Date: _____

Breakfast: _____ Lunch: _____

Dinner: _____ Snack: _____

Group	Fruits	Vegetables	Grains	Meat & Beans	Milk	Oils
Goal Amount						
Estimate Your Total						
Increase ⇧ or Decrease? ⇩						

Physical Activity: _____ Spiritual Activity: _____

Steps/Miles/Minutes: _____ _____

Day/Date: _____

Breakfast: _____ Lunch: _____

Dinner: _____ Snack: _____

Group	Fruits	Vegetables	Grains	Meat & Beans	Milk	Oils
Goal Amount						
Estimate Your Total						
Increase ⇧ or Decrease? ⇩						

Physical Activity: _____ Spiritual Activity: _____

Steps/Miles/Minutes: _____ _____

Day/Date: _____

Breakfast: _____ Lunch: _____

Dinner: _____ Snack: _____

Group	Fruits	Vegetables	Grains	Meat & Beans	Milk	Oils
Goal Amount						
Estimate Your Total						
Increase ⇧ or Decrease? ⇩						

Physical Activity: _____ Spiritual Activity: _____

Steps/Miles/Minutes: _____ _____

Live It Tracker

Name: _____ Loss/gain: _____ lbs.

Date: _____ Week #: _____ Calorie Range: _____ My food goal for next week: _____

Activity Level: None, < 30 min/day, 30-60 min/day, 60+ min/day My activity goal for next week: _____

Group	Daily Calories							
	1300-1400	1500-1600	1700-1800	1900-2000	2100-2200	2300-2400	2500-2600	2700-2800
Fruits	1.5-2 c.	1.5-2 c.	1.5-2 c.	2-2.5 c.	2-2.5 c.	2.5-3.5 c.	3.5-4.5 c.	3.5-4.5 c.
Vegetables	1.5-2 c.	2-2.5 c.	2.5-3 c.	2.5-3 c.	3-3.5 c.	3.5-4.5 c.	4.5-5 c.	4.5-5 c.
Grains	5 oz-eq.	5-6 oz-eq.	6-7 oz-eq.	6-7 oz-eq.	7-8 oz-eq.	8-9 oz-eq.	9-10 oz-eq.	10-11 oz-eq.
Meat & Beans	4 oz-eq.	5 oz-eq.	5-5.5 oz-eq.	5.5-6.5 oz-eq.	6.5-7 oz-eq.	7-7.5 oz-eq.	7-7.5 oz-eq.	7.5-8 oz-eq.
Milk	2-3 c.	3 c.	3 c.	3 c.	3 c.	3 c.	3 c.	3 c.
Healthy Oils	4 tsp.	5 tsp.	5 tsp.	6 tsp.	6 tsp.	7 tsp.	8 tsp.	8 tsp.

Day/Date:

Breakfast: _____ Lunch: _____

Dinner: _____ Snack: _____

Group	Fruits	Vegetables	Grains	Meat & Beans	Milk	Oils
Goal Amount						
Estimate Your Total						
Increase ⇧ or Decrease? ⇩						

Physical Activity: _____ Spiritual Activity: _____

Steps/Miles/Minutes: _____ _____

Day/Date:

Breakfast: _____ Lunch: _____

Dinner: _____ Snack: _____

Group	Fruits	Vegetables	Grains	Meat & Beans	Milk	Oils
Goal Amount						
Estimate Your Total						
Increase ⇧ or Decrease? ⇩						

Physical Activity: _____ Spiritual Activity: _____

Steps/Miles/Minutes: _____ _____

Day/Date:

Breakfast: _____ Lunch: _____

Dinner: _____ Snack: _____

Group	Fruits	Vegetables	Grains	Meat & Beans	Milk	Oils
Goal Amount						
Estimate Your Total						
Increase ⇧ or Decrease? ⇩						

Physical Activity: _____ Spiritual Activity: _____

Steps/Miles/Minutes: _____ _____

Day/Date: _____

Breakfast: _____ Lunch: _____

Dinner: _____ Snack: _____

Group	Fruits	Vegetables	Grains	Meat & Beans	Milk	Oils
Goal Amount						
Estimate Your Total						
Increase ⇧ or Decrease? ⇩						

Physical Activity: _____ Spiritual Activity: _____

Steps/Miles/Minutes: _____ _____

Day/Date: _____

Breakfast: _____ Lunch: _____

Dinner: _____ Snack: _____

Group	Fruits	Vegetables	Grains	Meat & Beans	Milk	Oils
Goal Amount						
Estimate Your Total						
Increase ⇧ or Decrease? ⇩						

Physical Activity: _____ Spiritual Activity: _____

Steps/Miles/Minutes: _____ _____

Day/Date: _____

Breakfast: _____ Lunch: _____

Dinner: _____ Snack: _____

Group	Fruits	Vegetables	Grains	Meat & Beans	Milk	Oils
Goal Amount						
Estimate Your Total						
Increase ⇧ or Decrease? ⇩						

Physical Activity: _____ Spiritual Activity: _____

Steps/Miles/Minutes: _____ _____

Day/Date: _____

Breakfast: _____ Lunch: _____

Dinner: _____ Snack: _____

Group	Fruits	Vegetables	Grains	Meat & Beans	Milk	Oils
Goal Amount						
Estimate Your Total						
Increase ⇧ or Decrease? ⇩						

Physical Activity: _____ Spiritual Activity: _____

Steps/Miles/Minutes: _____ _____

Live It Tracker

Name: _____ Loss/gain: _____ lbs.

Date: _____ Week #: _____ Calorie Range: _____ My food goal for next week: _____

Activity Level: None, < 30 min/day, 30-60 min/day, 60+ min/day My activity goal for next week: _____

Group	Daily Calories							
	1300-1400	1500-1600	1700-1800	1900-2000	2100-2200	2300-2400	2500-2600	2700-2800
Fruits	1.5-2 c.	1.5-2 c.	1.5-2 c.	2-2.5 c.	2-2.5 c.	2.5-3.5 c.	3.5-4.5 c.	3.5-4.5 c.
Vegetables	1.5-2 c.	2-2.5 c.	2.5-3 c.	2.5-3 c.	3-3.5 c.	3.5-4.5 c.	4.5-5 c.	4.5-5 c.
Grains	5 oz-eq.	5-6 oz-eq.	6-7 oz-eq.	6-7 oz-eq.	7-8 oz-eq.	8-9 oz-eq.	9-10 oz-eq.	10-11 oz-eq.
Meat & Beans	4 oz-eq.	5 oz-eq.	5-5.5 oz-eq.	5.5-6.5 oz-eq.	6.5-7 oz-eq.	7-7.5 oz-eq.	7-7.5 oz-eq.	7.5-8 oz-eq.
Milk	2-3 c.	3 c.	3 c.	3 c.	3 c.	3 c.	3 c.	3 c.
Healthy Oils	4 tsp.	5 tsp.	5 tsp.	6 tsp.	6 tsp.	7 tsp.	8 tsp.	8 tsp.

Day/Date:

Breakfast: _____ Lunch: _____

Dinner: _____ Snack: _____

Group	Fruits	Vegetables	Grains	Meat & Beans	Milk	Oils
Goal Amount						
Estimate Your Total						
Increase ⇧ or Decrease? ⇩						

Physical Activity: _____ Spiritual Activity: _____

Steps/Miles/Minutes: _____ _____

Day/Date:

Breakfast: _____ Lunch: _____

Dinner: _____ Snack: _____

Group	Fruits	Vegetables	Grains	Meat & Beans	Milk	Oils
Goal Amount						
Estimate Your Total						
Increase ⇧ or Decrease? ⇩						

Physical Activity: _____ Spiritual Activity: _____

Steps/Miles/Minutes: _____ _____

Day/Date:

Breakfast: _____ Lunch: _____

Dinner: _____ Snack: _____

Group	Fruits	Vegetables	Grains	Meat & Beans	Milk	Oils
Goal Amount						
Estimate Your Total						
Increase ⇧ or Decrease? ⇩						

Physical Activity: _____ Spiritual Activity: _____

Steps/Miles/Minutes: _____

Day/Date: _____

Breakfast: _____ Lunch: _____
_____
Dinner: _____ Snack: _____
_____

Group	Fruits	Vegetables	Grains	Meat & Beans	Milk	Oils
Goal Amount						
Estimate Your Total						
Increase ⇧ or Decrease? ⇩						

Physical Activity: _____ Spiritual Activity: _____

Steps/Miles/Minutes: _____ _____

Day/Date: _____

Breakfast: _____ Lunch: _____
_____
Dinner: _____ Snack: _____
_____

Group	Fruits	Vegetables	Grains	Meat & Beans	Milk	Oils
Goal Amount						
Estimate Your Total						
Increase ⇧ or Decrease? ⇩						

Physical Activity: _____ Spiritual Activity: _____

Steps/Miles/Minutes: _____ _____

Day/Date: _____

Breakfast: _____ Lunch: _____
_____
Dinner: _____ Snack: _____
_____

Group	Fruits	Vegetables	Grains	Meat & Beans	Milk	Oils
Goal Amount						
Estimate Your Total						
Increase ⇧ or Decrease? ⇩						

Physical Activity: _____ Spiritual Activity: _____

Steps/Miles/Minutes: _____ _____

Day/Date: _____

Breakfast: _____ Lunch: _____
_____
Dinner: _____ Snack: _____
_____

Group	Fruits	Vegetables	Grains	Meat & Beans	Milk	Oils
Goal Amount						
Estimate Your Total						
Increase ⇧ or Decrease? ⇩						

Physical Activity: _____ Spiritual Activity: _____

Steps/Miles/Minutes: _____ _____

Live It Tracker

Name: _____ Loss/gain: _____ lbs.

Date: _____ Week #: _____ Calorie Range: _____ My food goal for next week: _____

Activity Level: None, < 30 min/day, 30-60 min/day, 60+ min/day   My activity goal for next week: _____

Group	Daily Calories							
	1300-1400	1500-1600	1700-1800	1900-2000	2100-2200	2300-2400	2500-2600	2700-2800
Fruits	1.5-2 c.	1.5-2 c.	1.5-2 c.	2-2.5 c.	2-2.5 c.	2.5-3.5 c.	3.5-4.5 c.	3.5-4.5 c.
Vegetables	1.5-2 c.	2-2.5 c.	2.5-3 c.	2.5-3 c.	3-3.5 c.	3.5-4.5 c.	4.5-5 c.	4.5-5 c.
Grains	5 oz-eq.	5-6 oz-eq.	6-7 oz-eq.	6-7 oz-eq.	7-8 oz-eq.	8-9 oz-eq.	9-10 oz-eq.	10-11 oz-eq.
Meat & Beans	4 oz-eq.	5 oz-eq.	5-5.5 oz-eq.	5.5-6.5 oz-eq.	6.5-7 oz-eq.	7-7.5 oz-eq.	7-7.5 oz-eq.	7.5-8 oz-eq.
Milk	2-3 c.	3 c.	3 c.	3 c.	3 c.	3 c.	3 c.	3 c.
Healthy Oils	4 tsp.	5 tsp.	5 tsp.	6 tsp.	6 tsp.	7 tsp.	8 tsp.	8 tsp.

Breakfast: _____   Lunch: _____

Dinner: _____   Snack: _____

Group	Fruits	Vegetables	Grains	Meat & Beans	Milk	Oils
Goal Amount						
Estimate Your Total						
Increase ⬆ or Decrease? ⬇						

Physical Activity: _____   Spiritual Activity: _____

Steps/Miles/Minutes: _____

Breakfast: _____   Lunch: _____

Dinner: _____   Snack: _____

Group	Fruits	Vegetables	Grains	Meat & Beans	Milk	Oils
Goal Amount						
Estimate Your Total						
Increase ⬆ or Decrease? ⬇						

Physical Activity: _____   Spiritual Activity: _____

Steps/Miles/Minutes: _____

Breakfast: _____   Lunch: _____

Dinner: _____   Snack: _____

Group	Fruits	Vegetables	Grains	Meat & Beans	Milk	Oils
Goal Amount						
Estimate Your Total						
Increase ⬆ or Decrease? ⬇						

Physical Activity: _____   Spiritual Activity: _____

Steps/Miles/Minutes: _____

Day/Date: _____

Breakfast: _____ Lunch: _____

Dinner: _____ Snack: _____

Group	Fruits	Vegetables	Grains	Meat & Beans	Milk	Oils
Goal Amount						
Estimate Your Total						
Increase ⇧ or Decrease? ⇩						

Physical Activity: _____ Spiritual Activity: _____

Steps/Miles/Minutes: _____

Day/Date: _____

Breakfast: _____ Lunch: _____

Dinner: _____ Snack: _____

Group	Fruits	Vegetables	Grains	Meat & Beans	Milk	Oils
Goal Amount						
Estimate Your Total						
Increase ⇧ or Decrease? ⇩						

Physical Activity: _____ Spiritual Activity: _____

Steps/Miles/Minutes: _____

Day/Date: _____

Breakfast: _____ Lunch: _____

Dinner: _____ Snack: _____

Group	Fruits	Vegetables	Grains	Meat & Beans	Milk	Oils
Goal Amount						
Estimate Your Total						
Increase ⇧ or Decrease? ⇩						

Physical Activity: _____ Spiritual Activity: _____

Steps/Miles/Minutes: _____

Day/Date: _____

Breakfast: _____ Lunch: _____

Dinner: _____ Snack: _____

Group	Fruits	Vegetables	Grains	Meat & Beans	Milk	Oils
Goal Amount						
Estimate Your Total						
Increase ⇧ or Decrease? ⇩						

Physical Activity: _____ Spiritual Activity: _____

Steps/Miles/Minutes: _____

Live It Tracker

Name: _____ Loss/gain: _____ lbs.

Date: _____ Week #: _____ Calorie Range: _____ My food goal for next week: _____

Activity Level: None, < 30 min/day, 30-60 min/day, 60+ min/day   My activity goal for next week: _____

Group	Daily Calories							
	1300-1400	1500-1600	1700-1800	1900-2000	2100-2200	2300-2400	2500-2600	2700-2800
Fruits	1.5-2 c.	1.5-2 c.	1.5-2 c.	2-2.5 c.	2-2.5 c.	2.5-3.5 c.	3.5-4.5 c.	3.5-4.5 c.
Vegetables	1.5-2 c.	2-2.5 c.	2.5-3 c.	2.5-3 c.	3-3.5 c.	3.5-4.5 c.	4.5-5 c.	4.5-5 c.
Grains	5 oz-eq.	5-6 oz-eq.	6-7 oz-eq.	6-7 oz-eq.	7-8 oz-eq.	8-9 oz-eq.	9-10 oz-eq.	10-11 oz-eq.
Meat & Beans	4 oz-eq.	5 oz-eq.	5-5.5 oz-eq.	5.5-6.5 oz-eq.	6.5-7 oz-eq.	7-7.5 oz-eq.	7-7.5 oz-eq.	7.5-8 oz-eq.
Milk	2-3 c.	3 c.	3 c.	3 c.	3 c.	3 c.	3 c.	3 c.
Healthy Oils	4 tsp.	5 tsp.	5 tsp.	6 tsp.	6 tsp.	7 tsp.	8 tsp.	8 tsp.

Day/Date:

Breakfast: _____   Lunch: _____

Dinner: _____   Snack: _____

Group	Fruits	Vegetables	Grains	Meat & Beans	Milk	Oils
Goal Amount						
Estimate Your Total						
Increase ⇧ or Decrease? ⇩						

Physical Activity: _____   Spiritual Activity: _____

Steps/Miles/Minutes: _____

Day/Date:

Breakfast: _____   Lunch: _____

Dinner: _____   Snack: _____

Group	Fruits	Vegetables	Grains	Meat & Beans	Milk	Oils
Goal Amount						
Estimate Your Total						
Increase ⇧ or Decrease? ⇩						

Physical Activity: _____   Spiritual Activity: _____

Steps/Miles/Minutes: _____

Day/Date:

Breakfast: _____   Lunch: _____

Dinner: _____   Snack: _____

Group	Fruits	Vegetables	Grains	Meat & Beans	Milk	Oils
Goal Amount						
Estimate Your Total						
Increase ⇧ or Decrease? ⇩						

Physical Activity: _____   Spiritual Activity: _____

Steps/Miles/Minutes: _____

Day/Date: ___

Breakfast: _____ Lunch: _____

Dinner: _____ Snack: _____

Group	Fruits	Vegetables	Grains	Meat & Beans	Milk	Oils
Goal Amount						
Estimate Your Total						
Increase ⇧ or Decrease? ⇩						

Physical Activity: _____ Spiritual Activity: _____

Steps/Miles/Minutes: _____ _____

Day/Date: ___

Breakfast: _____ Lunch: _____

Dinner: _____ Snack: _____

Group	Fruits	Vegetables	Grains	Meat & Beans	Milk	Oils
Goal Amount						
Estimate Your Total						
Increase ⇧ or Decrease? ⇩						

Physical Activity: _____ Spiritual Activity: _____

Steps/Miles/Minutes: _____ _____

Day/Date: ___

Breakfast: _____ Lunch: _____

Dinner: _____ Snack: _____

Group	Fruits	Vegetables	Grains	Meat & Beans	Milk	Oils
Goal Amount						
Estimate Your Total						
Increase ⇧ or Decrease? ⇩						

Physical Activity: _____ Spiritual Activity: _____

Steps/Miles/Minutes: _____ _____

Day/Date: ___

Breakfast: _____ Lunch: _____

Dinner: _____ Snack: _____

Group	Fruits	Vegetables	Grains	Meat & Beans	Milk	Oils
Goal Amount						
Estimate Your Total						
Increase ⇧ or Decrease? ⇩						

Physical Activity: _____ Spiritual Activity: _____

Steps/Miles/Minutes: _____ _____

Live It Tracker

Name: _____ Loss/gain: _____ lbs.

Date: _____ Week #: _____ Calorie Range: _____ My food goal for next week: _____

Activity Level: None, < 30 min/day, 30-60 min/day, 60+ min/day My activity goal for next week: _____

Group	Daily Calories							
	1300-1400	1500-1600	1700-1800	1900-2000	2100-2200	2300-2400	2500-2600	2700-2800
Fruits	1.5-2 c.	1.5-2 c.	1.5-2 c.	2-2.5 c.	2-2.5 c.	2.5-3.5 c.	3.5-4.5 c.	3.5-4.5 c.
Vegetables	1.5-2 c.	2-2.5 c.	2.5-3 c.	2.5-3 c.	3-3.5 c.	3.5-4.5 c.	4.5-5 c.	4.5-5 c.
Grains	5 oz-eq.	5-6 oz-eq.	6-7 oz-eq.	6-7 oz-eq.	7-8 oz-eq.	8-9 oz-eq.	9-10 oz-eq.	10-11 oz-eq.
Meat & Beans	4 oz-eq.	5 oz-eq.	5-5.5 oz-eq.	5.5-6.5 oz-eq.	6.5-7 oz-eq.	7-7.5 oz-eq.	7-7.5 oz-eq.	7.5-8 oz-eq.
Milk	2-3 c.	3 c.	3 c.	3 c.	3 c.	3 c.	3 c.	3 c.
Healthy Oils	4 tsp.	5 tsp.	5 tsp.	6 tsp.	6 tsp.	7 tsp.	8 tsp.	8 tsp.

Day/Date: _____

Breakfast: _____ Lunch: _____

Dinner: _____ Snack: _____

Group	Fruits	Vegetables	Grains	Meat & Beans	Milk	Oils
Goal Amount						
Estimate Your Total						
Increase ⇧ or Decrease? ⇩						

Physical Activity: _____ Spiritual Activity: _____

Steps/Miles/Minutes: _____

Day/Date: _____

Breakfast: _____ Lunch: _____

Dinner: _____ Snack: _____

Group	Fruits	Vegetables	Grains	Meat & Beans	Milk	Oils
Goal Amount						
Estimate Your Total						
Increase ⇧ or Decrease? ⇩						

Physical Activity: _____ Spiritual Activity: _____

Steps/Miles/Minutes: _____

Day/Date: _____

Breakfast: _____ Lunch: _____

Dinner: _____ Snack: _____

Group	Fruits	Vegetables	Grains	Meat & Beans	Milk	Oils
Goal Amount						
Estimate Your Total						
Increase ⇧ or Decrease? ⇩						

Physical Activity: _____ Spiritual Activity: _____

Steps/Miles/Minutes: _____

Breakfast: _____ Lunch: _____

Dinner: _____ Snack: _____

Group	Fruits	Vegetables	Grains	Meat & Beans	Milk	Oils
Goal Amount						
Estimate Your Total						
Increase ⬆ or Decrease? ⬇						

Physical Activity: _____ Spiritual Activity: _____

Steps/Miles/Minutes: _____

Breakfast: _____ Lunch: _____

Dinner: _____ Snack: _____

Group	Fruits	Vegetables	Grains	Meat & Beans	Milk	Oils
Goal Amount						
Estimate Your Total						
Increase ⬆ or Decrease? ⬇						

Physical Activity: _____ Spiritual Activity: _____

Steps/Miles/Minutes: _____

Breakfast: _____ Lunch: _____

Dinner: _____ Snack: _____

Group	Fruits	Vegetables	Grains	Meat & Beans	Milk	Oils
Goal Amount						
Estimate Your Total						
Increase ⬆ or Decrease? ⬇						

Physical Activity: _____ Spiritual Activity: _____

Steps/Miles/Minutes: _____

Breakfast: _____ Lunch: _____

Dinner: _____ Snack: _____

Group	Fruits	Vegetables	Grains	Meat & Beans	Milk	Oils
Goal Amount						
Estimate Your Total						
Increase ⬆ or Decrease? ⬇						

Physical Activity: _____ Spiritual Activity: _____

Steps/Miles/Minutes: _____

Live It Tracker

Name: _____ Loss/gain: _____ lbs.

Date: _____ Week #: ____ Calorie Range: _____ My food goal for next week: _____

Activity Level: None, < 30 min/day, 30-60 min/day, 60+ min/day My activity goal for next week: _____

Group	Daily Calories							
	1300-1400	1500-1600	1700-1800	1900-2000	2100-2200	2300-2400	2500-2600	2700-2800
Fruits	1.5-2 c.	1.5-2 c.	1.5-2 c.	2-2.5 c.	2-2.5 c.	2.5-3.5 c.	3.5-4.5 c.	3.5-4.5 c.
Vegetables	1.5-2 c.	2-2.5 c.	2.5-3 c.	2.5-3 c.	3-3.5 c.	3.5-4.5 c.	4.5-5 c.	4.5-5 c.
Grains	5 oz-eq.	5-6 oz-eq.	6-7 oz-eq.	6-7 oz-eq.	7-8 oz-eq.	8-9 oz-eq.	9-10 oz-eq.	10-11 oz-eq.
Meat & Beans	4 oz-eq.	5 oz-eq.	5-5.5 oz-eq.	5.5-6.5 oz-eq.	6.5-7 oz-eq.	7-7.5 oz-eq.	7-7.5 oz-eq.	7.5-8 oz-eq.
Milk	2-3 c.	3 c.	3 c.	3 c.	3 c.	3 c.	3 c.	3 c.
Healthy Oils	4 tsp.	5 tsp.	5 tsp.	6 tsp.	6 tsp.	7 tsp.	8 tsp.	8 tsp.

Day/Date: _____

Breakfast: _____ Lunch: _____

Dinner: _____ Snack: _____

Group	Fruits	Vegetables	Grains	Meat & Beans	Milk	Oils
Goal Amount						
Estimate Your Total						
Increase ⇧ or Decrease? ⇩						

Physical Activity: _____ Spiritual Activity: _____

Steps/Miles/Minutes: _____

Day/Date: _____

Breakfast: _____ Lunch: _____

Dinner: _____ Snack: _____

Group	Fruits	Vegetables	Grains	Meat & Beans	Milk	Oils
Goal Amount						
Estimate Your Total						
Increase ⇧ or Decrease? ⇩						

Physical Activity: _____ Spiritual Activity: _____

Steps/Miles/Minutes: _____

Day/Date: _____

Breakfast: _____ Lunch: _____

Dinner: _____ Snack: _____

Group	Fruits	Vegetables	Grains	Meat & Beans	Milk	Oils
Goal Amount						
Estimate Your Total						
Increase ⇧ or Decrease? ⇩						

Physical Activity: _____ Spiritual Activity: _____

Steps/Miles/Minutes: _____

Day/Date: _____

Breakfast: _____   Lunch: _____
_____

Dinner: _____   Snack: _____
_____

Group	Fruits	Vegetables	Grains	Meat & Beans	Milk	Oils
Goal Amount						
Estimate Your Total						
Increase ⇧ or Decrease? ⇩						

Physical Activity: _____   Spiritual Activity: _____
Steps/Miles/Minutes: _____   _____

Day/Date: _____

Breakfast: _____   Lunch: _____
_____

Dinner: _____   Snack: _____
_____

Group	Fruits	Vegetables	Grains	Meat & Beans	Milk	Oils
Goal Amount						
Estimate Your Total						
Increase ⇧ or Decrease? ⇩						

Physical Activity: _____   Spiritual Activity: _____
Steps/Miles/Minutes: _____   _____

Day/Date: _____

Breakfast: _____   Lunch: _____
_____

Dinner: _____   Snack: _____
_____

Group	Fruits	Vegetables	Grains	Meat & Beans	Milk	Oils
Goal Amount						
Estimate Your Total						
Increase ⇧ or Decrease? ⇩						

Physical Activity: _____   Spiritual Activity: _____
Steps/Miles/Minutes: _____   _____

Day/Date: _____

Breakfast: _____   Lunch: _____
_____

Dinner: _____   Snack: _____
_____

Group	Fruits	Vegetables	Grains	Meat & Beans	Milk	Oils
Goal Amount						
Estimate Your Total						
Increase ⇧ or Decrease? ⇩						

Physical Activity: _____   Spiritual Activity: _____
Steps/Miles/Minutes: _____   _____

let's count our miles!

Join the 100-Mile Club this Session

Can't walk that mile yet? Don't be discouraged! There are exercises you can do to strengthen your body and burn those extra calories. Keep a record on your Live It Tracker of the number of minutes you do these common physical activities, convert those minutes to miles following the chart below, and then mark off each mile you have completed on the chart found on the back of the front cover. Report your miles to your 100-Mile Club representative when you first arrive each week. Remember, you are not competing with anyone else . . . just yourself. Your job is to strive to reach 100 miles before the last meeting in this session. You can do it—just keep on moving!

Walking

slowly, 2 mph	30 min. = 156 cal. = 1 mile
moderately, 3 mph	20 min. = 156 cal. = 1 mile
very briskly, 4 mph	15 min. = 156 cal. = 1 mile
speed walking	10 min. = 156 cal. = 1 mile
up stairs	13 min. = 159 cal. = 1 mile

Running/Jogging

10 min. = 156 cal. = 1 mile

Cycling Outdoors

slowly, <10 mph	20 min. = 156 cal. = 1 mile
light effort, 10-12 mph	12 min. = 156 cal. = 1 mile
moderate effort, 12-14 mph.	10 min. = 156 cal. = 1 mile
vigorous effort, 14-16 mph	7.5 min. = 156 cal. = 1 mile
very fast, 16-19 mph	6.5 min. = 152 cal. = 1 mile

Sports Activities

Playing tennis (singles)	10 min. = 156 cal. = 1 mile
Swimming	
light to moderate effort	11 min. = 152 cal. = 1 mile
fast, vigorous effort	7.5 min. = 156 cal. = 1 mile
Softball	15 min. = 156 cal. = 1 mile
Golf	20 min. = 156 cal = 1 mile
Rollerblading	6.5 min. = 152 cal. = 1 mile
Ice skating	11 min. = 152 cal. = 1 mile

Jumping rope	7.5 min. = 156 cal. = 1 mile
Basketball	12 min. = 156 cal. = 1 mile
Soccer (casual)	15 min. = 159 cal. = 1 mile

Around the House

Mowing grass	22 min. = 156 cal. = 1 mile
Mopping, sweeping, vacuuming	19.5 min. = 155 cal. = 1 mile
Cooking	40 min. =160 cal. = 1 mile
Gardening	19 min. = 156 cal. = 1 mile
Housework (general)	35 min. = 156 cal. = 1 mile
Ironing	45 min. = 153 cal. = 1 mile
Raking leaves	25 min. = 150 cal. = 1 mile
Washing car	23 min. = 156 cal. = 1 mile
Washing dishes	45 min. = 153 cal. = 1 mile

At the Gym

Stair machine	8.5 min. = 155 cal. = 1 mile
Stationary bike	
slowly, 10 mph	30 min. = 156 cal. = 1 mile
moderately, 10-13 mph	15 min. = 156 cal. = 1 mile
vigorously, 13-16 mph	7.5 min. = 156 cal. = 1 mile
briskly, 16-19 mph	6.5 min. = 156 cal. = 1 mile
Elliptical trainer	12 min. = 156 cal. = 1 mile
Weight machines (used vigorously)	13 min. = 152 cal.=1 mile
Aerobics	
low impact	15 min. = 156 cal. = 1 mile
high impact	12 min. = 156 cal. = 1 mile
water	20 min. = 156 cal. = 1 mile
Pilates	15 min. = 156 cal. = 1 mile
Raquetball (casual)	15 min. = 159 cal. = 1 mile
Stretching exercises	25 min. = 150 cal. = 1 mile
Weight lifting (also works for weight machines used moderately or gently)	30 min. = 156 cal. = 1 mile

Family Leisure

Playing piano	37 min. = 155 cal. = 1 mile
Jumping rope	10 min. = 152 cal. = 1 mile
Skating (moderate)	20 min. = 152 cal. = 1 mile
Swimming	
moderate	17 min. = 156 cal. = 1 mile
vigorous	10 min. = 148 cal. = 1 mile
Table tennis	25 min. = 150 cal. = 1 mile
Walk/run/play with kids	25 min. = 150 cal. = 1 mile

Week 2: Relying on His Goodness

Restore to me the joy of your salvation and grant me a willing spirit, to sustain me.

Week 3: Convinced of His love

May the God of hope fill you with all joy and peace as you trust in him, so that you may overflow with hope by the power of the Holy Spirit.

Giving Christ Control

Giving Christ Control
Scripture Memory Verses:

PSALM 51:12   ROMANS 12:3
ROMANS 15:13   JAMES 1:26
PHILIPPIANS 4:8   LUKE 9:23
GALATIANS 2:20   HEBREWS 10:24-25
PHILIPPIANS 4:12-13   1 THESSALONIANS 5:23

How to Use These Cards:

Separate cards from the Bible study book. These cards are designed to be used when exercising. To do this, you may want to punch a hole in the upper left corner of the cards and place on a ring. When you have finished memorizing all the verses from one study, add the new Bible study cards to the ring and continue practicing the old verses while learning the new ones. Cards may be placed anywhere you will see them regularly—on the dashboard of your car, on a mirror, on a desk. After you have memorized the verse, begin using the reverse side of the card so the reference is connected to the verse. This is a great way to practice the verses you have already learned.

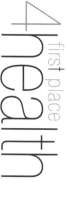

first place 4health

discover a new way to healthy living

Psalm 51:12

Romans 15:13

Week 6: Yielding Our Desires

I have learned the secret of being content in any and every situation, whether well fed or hungry, whether living in plenty or in want. I can do everything through him who gives me strength.

Week 7: Releasing Our Calling

Do not think of yourself more highly than you ought, but rather think of yourself with sober judgment, in accordance with the measure of faith God has given you.

Week 4: Yielding to His Glory

Finally, brothers, whatever is true, whatever is noble, whatever is right, whatever is pure, whatever is lovely, whatever is admirable—if anything is excellent or praiseworthy— think about such things.

Week 5: Control: Whose Reponsibility Is It?

I have been crucified with Christ and I no longer live, but Christ lives in me. The life I live in the body, I live by faith in the Son of God, who loved me and gave himself for me.

PHILIPPIANS 4:12-13

PHILIPPIANS 4:8

ROMANS 12:3

GALATIANS 2:20

Week 8: Surrendering Our Words

If anyone considers himself religious and yet does not keep a tight rein on his tongue, he deceives himself and his religion is worthless.

Week 9: How to Let Go of Control

If anyone would come after me, he must deny himself and take up his cross daily and follow me.

Week 10: A Community of Encouragement

Let us consider how we may spur one another on toward love and good deeds. Let us not give up meeting together, as some are in the habit of doing, but let us encourage one another—and all the more as you see the Day approaching.

Week 11: A Life of Purpose

May God himself, the God of peace, sanctify you through and through. May your whole spirit, soul and body be kept blameless at the coming of our Lord Jesus Christ.

HEBREWS 10:24-25

JAMES 1:26

1 THESSALONIANS 5:23

LUKE 9:23